AROMATHERAPY

Dedication

I would like to dedicate this book to my beloved father, Dr Hugo Lenart, who let me share his love of Medicine, Nature and Healing, and to Hugo and Andrew, my wonderful sons, and Bill, my husband and partner.

THE AUTHOR

Dr Vivian Nadya Lunny is recognized as an expert in the field of Aromatherapy. She is co-founder, co-principal and director of The International Academy of Holistic Studies in Great Britain. She specializes in clinical consultancy, and professional and individualized patient treatments in aromatherapy, color therapy, and stress management. She is an international conference speaker, seminar presenter, and workshop leader and travels extensively, lecturing and undertaking research programs. She has had several articles and scientific research papers published dealing with aromatherapy related topics.

The Institute for Complementary Medicine

The Institute for Complementary Medicine (ICM) was founded in Britain in 1982. It is a charitable organization whose aim is to encourage the development of all forms of complementary medicine, including research, education, and standards of clinical practice, and to provide factual information to the Media and the public. With over 370 affiliated organizations, the ICM sees complementary medicine as a separate and independent source of health care, yet it always encourages a correct relationship with the medical profession to ensure each case receives the most appropriate treatment available.

COMPLEMENTARY HEALTH

AROMATHERAPY

VIVIAN LUNNY M.D.

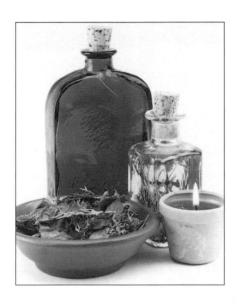

SMITHMARK

A Salamander Book

© Salamander Books Ltd., 1997.
129–137 York Way,
London N7 9LG,
United Kingdom.

This edition published in 1997 by SMITHMARK Publishers,
a division of U.S. Media Holdings, Inc.,
16 East 32nd Street,
New York, NY 10016.

9 8 7 6 5 4 3 2 1

SMITHMARK books are available for bulk purchase for sales promotion
and premium use. For details write or call the manager of special sales,
SMITHMARK Publishers,
16 East 32nd Street,
New York,
NY 10016; (212) 532–6600

ISBN 0–7651–9955–6

This book was created by SP Creative Design for Salamander Books Ltd.
Editor: Heather Thomas
Designer: Al Rockall
Production: Rolando Ugolini
Illustration reproduction: Emirates Printing Press, Dubai
Printed in Spain

Photography:
Studio photography by Bruce Head

IMPORTANT

The information, recipes and remedies contained in this book are
generally applicable and appropriate in most cases, but are not tailored to
specific circumstances or individuals. The authors and publishers cannot
be held responsible for any problems arising from the mistaken identity of
any plants or remedies, or the inappropriate use of any remedy or recipe.
Do not undertake any form of self diagnosis or treatment for serious
complaints without first seeking professional advice. Always seek
professional medical advice if symptoms persist.

CONTENTS

CHAPTER ONE

THE WORLD OF SCENTS AND AROMATHERAPY

Aromatherapy is a complete psychosomatic system of healing, a holistic approach to health and well-being by means of aromas—scents derived from the plant kingdom. It can be described as an art as well as a science; an art because of the intuitive, creative and esthetic aspects of preparing special blends for each individual person, and a science because it rests on sound scientific knowledge.

The use of aromatic substances in healing, far from being a newly-discovered therapy, has been with mankind since the beginning of time. There is not only anecdotal but also practical evidence of the use of plant essences by many ancient civilizations all over our planet.

CHINA, INDIA AND JAPAN

The Chinese were amongst the first to discover and use the medicinal properties of plants. This medical knowledge goes back to the third millennium B.C. when the Emperor Chen Nang (circa 2800B.C.) in his book *Pen Tsao* revealed the usage of no less than 100 plants, including Aniseed, Canela, Ginger, and Curcuma.

In traditional Indian Ayurvedic Medicine, the sacred book, thought to have been produced by Brahma, revealed that the secret of long life was related to the use of aromatic plants not only as food but also as medicine. The first known medicinal oil was that extracted from the Neem tree of India; many parts of the tree have been used since at least 4000B.C. and the spiritual association made with it is clear from the Harappan seals of the Indus Valley civilization. The Attar of Rose, essence of rose, is thought to have been discovered by the Indian Empress Nur Jehan Begum, in 1612.

ANCIENT EGYPT

In Egypt, from about 4236B.C., the first year of their calendar, to 30B.C., the use of aromatic plants went through some considerable changes. At the beginning, only pharaohs were considered close enough to the Divine to use essences which were kept by the priests. Around 2450B.C., Phan Hotep was telling Egyptian men the proper way to conduct their marriages: "If thou art a man of standing thou shouldst fill her belly, clothe her back and ointment is the prescription of her body." Plant substances were transported by large caravans and commanded gold prices—amongst them Cedarwood from the Lebanon, Myrrh from Ethiopia and Somalia, Roses from Damascus, Labdanum and Nard.

Immenohthep, the famous architect of the Saqqarah Pyramid, physician of the third dynasty to Pharaoh Djoser, was famed throughout the ancient world for his wisdom and great knowledge of medicine. He is said to have obtained his medicines by using aromatic plants—mainly Aniseed, Cinnamon, Cardamom, Cumin and Olibanum. In later dynasties, he was known as Ptah-Hotep, and his pyramid as the step pyramid. The Egyptians mastered the production of aromatic products, such as floral waters, cosmetic products, preparations destined for embalming, ceremonial oils, ointments, and odoriferous resins symbolic of the Eternal Way.

BABYLONIANS AND HEBREWS

The aristocrats of ancient Babylon believed that at palace banquets the aroma was as important an element as the food. Guests would have their individual "cassoulette," incense burner, at their place setting.

The Hebrews inherited their practices from the Egyptians and put great emphasis on personal hygiene. In the Bible, Proverbs 27:9, we are told, "Ointment and perfume rejoice the heart: so doth the sweetness of a man's friend by

hearty counsel." And in Revelations 5:8 it says "that vials full of odours are the prayers of Saints." In the book of Exodus, Jehovah gave Moses the formulation of an incense and an anointing oil destined for divine service.

King Solomon (960B.C.) had his famous Temple in Jerusalem built of Lebanon Cedar wood and stone. Precious Myrrh and incense were two of the three Wise Men's offerings to the new-born Jesus. Frankincense is a profoundly spiritual oil and Myrrh is a healing agent due to its anti-bacterial properties.

PHOENICIANS AND GREEKS

Phoenician merchants brought back from their trips to the Orient Cinnamon, Frankincense, Ginger and Myrrh.

Esculapius, god and king of Thesalia,

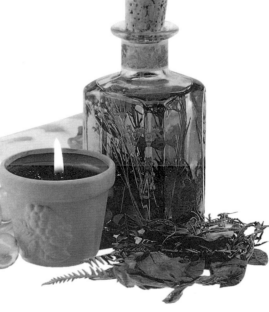

Right: essential oils and aromatherapy products can be used for health and beauty.

was a renowned physician. His two daughters Hygeia and Panaceae have always represented the two main approaches to therapeutics: Hygeia, the goddess ruler of Preservation of Health, and Panaceae, the goddess ruler of Curative Medicine.

Along these lines Hippocrates of Cos (460–377B.C.) compiled all the medical knowledge of his time in 72 books called *Corpus Hippocraticum.* In separating illness from the magical, he recognized natural influences and proposed a basic principle of natural forces. Hippocrates recommended the use of aromatics for use as food and medicine, as well as a fragrant massage every day for good health.

Galen (A.D.130–200), physician to several Roman emperors, contributed a great deal to the history of pharmacology. Galen's method of prescribing pays homage to its originator who provided a reference for the practicing physician.

NORTH AND SOUTH AMERICA

The Incas, Aztecs and Mayans possessed a perfect knowledge of their regional medicinal plants as well as drugs and toxic plants. Traditional medicine possessed empirical knowledge which science later confirmed.

Right: the essential oils are mixed with carrier oils.

Research into the efficacy of aromatic plants confirmed their traditional usage in 80 percent of cases.

Since antiquity native people have utilized resins naturally, extracting them from trees for the treatment of infections and other various lesions. Amongst them are Copaiba Balsam from the Amazon (used for countless poultices), Tolu Balsam, Peru Balsam, Sassafras, Rosewood and Guaiac Wood.

Indigenous North American tribes also had a wealth of knowledge of plant medicines, many of which were adopted by the first settlers in America. Plants, such as Sweet Grass and Sage Bush, were used not only as medicines but also as sacred and ceremonial incenses.

EVOLUTION OF AROMATHERAPY

Avicenna, a Persian poet, philosopher,

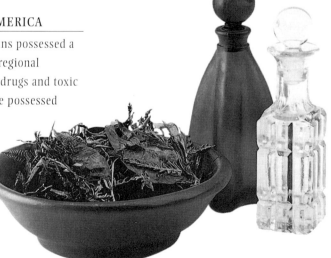

scholar and physician, wrote his *Canon of Medicine* around the year 1000 and re-established steam distillation. The earliest that we still have knowledge of was invented by an alchemist who worked in Italy during the third century known as "Maria Prophetissima."

Alchemy reached its peak with Teophrastus Bombastus von Hohenzolen, better known as Paracelsus. He was a famous sixteenth century physician, surgeon and chemist who established the correspondences between the Universe (macro-cosmos), and different parts of the human body (micro-cosmos).

The earliest scientific research into aromatic oils was carried out in France by Chamberland (1887) whose work was validated by Cadac and Meunier two years later. Martindale (1910) classified essential oils according to their antiseptic power related to their phenolic content.

R.M. Gattefossé, believed to have coined the term *Aromatherapie*, was a chemist. His story is aromatherapeutic history— he burnt his hand while conducting an experiment in his laboratory, and as a reflex action he immersed it in a nearby container which contained essential oil of Lavender. Gattefossé found the pain was lessened and the healing process more pronounced from this application of Lavender. The scientific papers and books of Gattefossé, Guenther, Gidlemeister and Hofman, Valnet, and their followers confirmed the therapeutic value of essential oils.

SAFETY FIRST

There is a set of guidelines regarding the safe use of essential oils, not only by the professional aromatherapist but also by the lay reader. These should be followed strictly before embarking on the home use of aromatics and massage. The main guidelines are as follows:

■ Essential oils should not be used undiluted. However, in the hands of a clinically trained aromatherapist some oils may be used neat in very small quantities and over localized areas.

■ In the case of patients with cancer, massage should not be attempted. The only exception to this rule is when the therapist has undertaken specialized further training in the treatment of cancer sufferers.

■ Dosages for the elderly and the very young should be calculated according to those described in the relevant chapters.

■ Oils that are not pure, natural and derived from a known sole botanical source should not be used for treatments.

■ Do not massage anyone who is suffering from a high temperature, a skin infection, or any infectious childhood disease.

■ Do not use mineral oils as vehicles or carriers.

■ Do not massage when a person has recently had an accident without first consulting their doctor.

CHAPTER TWO

ESSENTIAL OILS

In this chapter, you will find a directory of some of the most commonly used essential oils with detailed information about the plant from which they where obtained, their therapeutic effects, and chemical constituents (for an explanation of the star system used, turn to page 65.) The ordinary layperson using essential oils does not need to study each oil's chemical constituents, but they are reproduced for your information and interest.

An essential oil is a conglomeration of energetic atoms. Essential oils are aromatic liquids contained within an aromatic plant. They are fragrant, highly volatile (quickly evaporating in contact with air) liquids which are produced naturally in specialized glands of aromatic plants as a part of the mechanism of photosynthesis. It is often said by complementary practitioners who use essential oils that they contain the life force of the plant. Indeed, some romantic botanists state that the fragrance of an essential oil is a plant's signature, while in literature essential oils are sometimes described as the life and soul of an aromatic plant. However, always remember that essential oils are very volatile and should be handled with respect and care.

Essential oils are produced in plants during the process of photosynthesis, which is part of the plant's metabolic cycle. Over the years, researchers have offered different theories about this. For example, perserite (a type of alcohol) and other polyhydric alcohols, which are found in aromatic plants and also contain over six hydroxylic functions, may be the foundations for the formation process of essential oils during photosynthesis.

PROPERTIES AND EFFECTS OF ESSENTIAL OILS

Essential oils have a unique effect due to the complexity of their chemical structure. An individual essential oil could contain approximately 230 or more distinct volatile molecules. It is because of their diffusibility that they can be placed amongst the healing plant resources for all living beings. The principal general advantages which can be gained by the use of essential oils can be summarized as follows:

■ Essential oils are used as a "whole" and pure plant essence; the appearance of side effects is greatly diminished, and hence their correct use is relatively safe.

■ Due to the transdermal diffusion of essential oils they can be applied easily to the epidermis (skin) to gain beneficial effects. Natural inhalation can also be used safely and effectively under direction.

■ Some essential oil-containing plants have traditionally been used in cookery, such as Garlic, Cardamom, and Caraway in Central and Northern Europe; Citronella in India; Ginger in China; Basil in Greece; and Oregano in Spain and Italy. It is this traditional use, along with indigenous medicinal use, combined with a century of scientific research and therapeutic successes, that has enabled us today to see the effectiveness of essential oils.

■ The oils with the strongest anti-infectious action known are those that are commonly found in cooking. These, for example, are Clove, Cinnamon, Oregano, Mountain Savoury, and Thyme, which possess the same or a higher action than any known preparatory antiseptic or disinfectant.

■ Essential oils in their structure have the potential to donate or receive electrons. This energetic exchange is due to the wavelength of the electromagnetic vibrations which are produced by the essential oils.

■ The recognized healing effect of essential oils is thought to be carried out mainly through tissue stimulation. This quality refers to the healing and regenerating action of certain essential oils.

■ Essential oils have an analgesic neutralizing effect upon the chemicals carried by the sensory dendrites (nerve endings) in response to injury. This is generally felt as pain and the effect of neutralization leads to the absence of pain or discomfort.

■ The anti-inflammatory effect is achieved by the inhibition of the local inflammatory response and neutralization of chemical reactions caused by an injury.

■ Essential oils act directly upon the hypothalamic (brain) centers, which have a regulating effect upon the pituitary gland known as the hypophysis, through hormones with the rest of the endocrine system. Some essential oils are able to regulate endocrine dysfunctions and immune disorders.

BENEFICIAL EFFECTS

Therefore we can conclude that essential oils have a great many beneficial effects upon all living beings, many of which are elusive. They are able to re-establish homeostasis (harmony), and balance or ground a person to achieve a state of equilibrium, in addition to restoring well-being through the body and mind connections.

Some essential oils, such as *Melaleuca alternifolia*, commonly known as Tea Tree, produce an increase in natural acidity, and efficiently balance organic alkalinity occurring in skin diseases, such as acne, and fungi as in the case of athlete's foot. It is believed that essential oils are indirectly able to neutralize extreme acidity by acting on the central nervous system.

Below: essential oils are always stored in well-stoppered dark glass bottles.

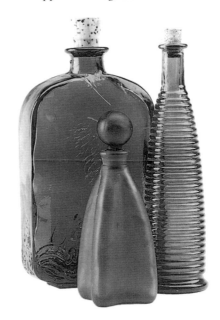

WHERE AND HOW DO WE GET THEM?

We gain our essential oils from diverse parts of aromatic plants.

■ **Roots and rhizomes** as in the case of *Vetiveria zizanoides*, commonly known as Vetiver, and *Zingiber officinalis* (Ginger).

■ **Fruits** as in the case of *Juniperus communis*, also known as Juniper.

■ **Buds** as in the case of *Eugenia caryophylata*, commonly known as Cloves.

■ **Leaves** such as *Rosmarinus officinalis*, commonly known as Rosemary, and *Thymus vulgaris* (Thyme).

■ **Petals** such as *Rosa damascena*, commonly known as Rose, and *Citrus aurantium* var. *amara*, also known as Neroli.

■ **Flowering heads** such as *Anthemis nobilis*, better known as Roman Chamomile, *Matricaria recutita*, commonly known as German Chamomile, and many others.

■ **Rind of citrus fruits** such as *Citrus bergamia*, known as Bergamot, and *Citrus limonum*, better known as Lemon.

■ **Resin** obtained from plants such as *Commiphora myrrha*, known as Myrrh, and *Boswellia carterii*, commonly known as Frankincense.

ENFLEURAGE

This is a method of non-volatile or fixed solvent extraction at normal temperatures based on the absorption of a flower fragrance by highly purified and odorless solid fat. In times past this fat used to be a closely-guarded secret by the distiller.

EXPRESSION

There are three main methods of expressed extraction, which is the most commonly used extraction method to extract the citrus oils from the peel of Lemon, Orange, Bergamot, Grapefruit, Mandarin, Lime, and other citrus fruits.

THE PROCESS OF DISTILLATION

This is simple distillation of plants and liquids at atmospheric pressure. The plant material and/or liquids to be distilled are placed in a distillation vessel. This vessel is fitted with a tube at or near its upper

EXTRACTION METHODS

The most commonly used methods to extract essential oils that are suitable for therapeutic use are:

■ Steam distillation
■ Water distillation
■ Expression
■ CO_2 (carbon dioxide) extraction
■ Natural solvent extraction

Distillation

The separation of volatile oils from plants and their flowers by distillation can, if carried out correctly, yield exceptionally good therapeutic quality essential oils. Distillation is the process of converting a volatile material into a vapor/steam, and then by condensing the vapor/steam by cooling, the fragrant or volatile substance can be separated and collected. In the case of essential oils, the separation occurs naturally due to their molecular weight.

section to enable the vapor to fall into a downward slope, or in a vertical water-cooled condenser. To enable this to happen the liquid has to be heated past the boiling point. This vapor/steam from the boiling liquid or plant material then passes into the cooling condenser where it condenses into a liquid. The condensed liquid is then collected in what is called a receiver flask.

The remaining distillation water, once it is separated from an essential oil, nearly always carries the fragrance of the oil, giving us evidence, to some extent, that some essential oil molecules are water soluble.

PURCHASING QUALITY CONTROL

In order to be assured of the quality of essential oils, the following points need to be carefully considered.

1 The botanical identity and origin of the plant's given essential oil, namely the family, genus, species and subspecies.

2 Information regarding the cultivation of the plant, the environment in which it grows and whether the harvesting of the plant material is done by hand or machine.

3 The option of purchasing a chemical profile or gas chromatography profile of the essential oil, which may be relevant when dealing with subspecies and chemotypes (variations naturally occurring within a plant when its habitat) is modified.

4 To get the finest therapeutic oil we should be informed by which method of extraction the essential oil has been gained. As we will see later on, there are specific methods of extraction which are applied to different plants.

LABELING OF ESSENTIAL OILS

Looking for 100 percent pure essential oils, the description and labeling of therapeutic essential oils should contain more than two of the following descriptive terms.

1 **Organically grown:** this refers to cultivated plants that should have been grown in pesticide-free soil. The term refers to the same condition laid down for vegetables, depending upon the country's soil associations. The plants should also not have been subject to synthetic pesticides.

2 **Wild grown:** this is a term that refers to the plant growing in its original, natural habitat and which has not been planted there by man, including:

■ The rainforest or at high altitude.

■ Mountainous areas, where it is not subject to known pollutants, or diverse atmospheric conditions.

3 **One hundred percent pure:** this refers to an unblended essential oil, which has not been recycled, bleached or colored. No other liquid substance should be present in the bottle of essential oil.

4 **One hundred percent natural:** without any additional synthetic substances.

ANTHEMIS NOBILIS OR CHAMOEMELUM NOBILE
Chamomile (Roman)

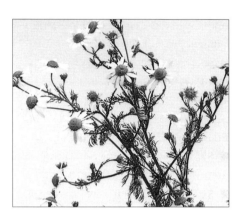

Anthemis nobilis or *Chamoemelum nobile* is also known by the names of English Chamomile, Lawn Camomile, *Manzanilla* (Spanish), *Kamilla* (Hungarian), *Kamille* (German) and *Chamille* (French). It belongs to the *Compositae*, also known as *Asteraceae*, family. Roman Chamomile is grown in Southern and Western Europe, England, Belgium, Chile, France, Hungary, Italy and the United States.

ESSENTIAL OIL

This is obtained by steam distillation of the flowering tops, which are hand-picked to ensure the best quality oil. It has been estimated that 132 pounds of flowering tops are needed to produce two pounds of essential oil.

It is a Middle Note oil, with a calming, soothing, mothering temperament. It has a fresh scent with a strongly herbaceous undertone and a very light blue or clear, pale yellow color, which turns to a stronger shade of yellow with age.

THE PLANT

The adult plant reaches only nine to 12 inches in height. It creeps or trails along the surface of the soil, with hairy stems which branch freely. The stems divide into fine, thread-like segments, giving the plant a feathery appearance. The blooms (from June to September) are solitary on erect stems, the outer radiated petals around a yellow center resembling a daisy. Each bloom has approximately eighteen rays, situated around a conical receptacle with yellow tubular florets. Between the florets are chaffy scales, which are short and blunt. The whole plant is downy and grayish green in appearance.

The ancient Egyptians revered this plant, relating it to the Sun God. The ancient Greeks called it "ground apple," and its name is probably derived from *kamai* (the Greek for "ground"). For hundreds of years, Chamomile has been regarded as a "small herb with vast healing powers," which brings solace to the wounded in body or spirit.

THERAPEUTIC EFFECTS

Negative charging molecules,

analgesic, anti-inflammatory, anesthetic (in pre-medication), anti-convulsive, anti-spasmodic, calming effect on the central nervous system, nervous tonic and sedative.

INDICATIONS AND COMMON USES

Therapeutic value ★ ★ ★ ★

PHYSICAL SPHERE

■ **Skeletal system:** the oil is beneficial for treating arthritis and chilblains.

■ **Skin:** beneficial for various types of dermatitis, eczema, psoriasis, sensitive and inflamed skin.

■ **Respiratory system:** useful for treating asthma triggered by stress.

■ **Peripheral nerves:** good for neuritis, the inflammation of the peripheral nerves and their endings.

■ **Teeth:** a recognized remedy for teething pains and toothache.

PSYCHO-SPIRITUAL SPHERE

Roman Chamomile is exceptional in treating anger, bed-wetting in children due to stress, children's temper tantrums, insomnia due to an over-active mind, stress, tension, and excessive worry.

 ## BLENDS WELL WITH

Bergamot, German Chamomile, True Lavender, Neroli, Rosewood, Sandalwood, Tea Tree.

CHEMICAL CONSTITUENTS OF ESSENTIAL OIL

ALCOHOLS:

■ Terpenic alcohols 5–6%: trans-pinocarveol, farnesol

ESTERS:

■ Alyphatic esters 75-80%

■ Butyrates: isoamyl butyrate 2.5%, isobutyl iso-butyrate, methyl–2 isobutyl butyrate, of metyl 1–2, 2 metyl-butyl butyrate, metyle 1–2 butyrate, isoamyl-methyl (1–2) – 3 metyl lpentalyl butyrate

■ Angelates: metacryl angelate, methyl angelate, butyl angelate, isobutyl angelate, 3 methyl 1 pentalyl angelate, butyl and propyl angelate, 2 methyl 2 propyl angelate

■ Isovalerates: butyl isovalerate, amyl isovalerate

■ Tiglates: isobutyl tiglate, isoamyl tiglate, methyl tiglate

METACHRILATES

CROTONATES

KETONES

■ Terpenic ketones: pinocarvone.
Lactones

■ Sesquiterpenic lactones: 3 deshydronobilene.

SAFETY PRECAUTIONS

None known at usual blending dosages.

BOSWELLIA CARTERII OR BOSWELLIA THURIFERA

Frankincense

Frankincense belongs to the *Burseraceae* family. It is mainly produced in Ethiopia, Somalia, China, Arabia, and India.

ESSENTIAL OIL

Native to Northeast Africa, the essential oil of Frankincense is obtained from the resinoid by steam distillation. It is a Base Note oil with a warming, soothing temperament, a warm, rich, balsamic scent, and a pale yellow to greenish color.

THE PLANT

A small tree or shrub with abundant pinnate leaves and pink flowers. The trees of the Somali coast grow without soil, out of rocks to which they are attached by a thick oval mass of a substance resembling a mixture of lime and mortar. The young trees yield the most valuable gum. A deep longitudinal incision is made on the trunk of the tree, and below it a narrow strip of bark, about four inches in length is peeled off. When the milk-like juice which it exudes has hardened by exposure to the air, the incision is deepened. In about three months the resin reaches the expected degree of consistency hardening into "yellowish tears."

Known since antiquity, the ceremonial incense of the Jews was made up of four sweet scents of which Frankincense was one. With other spices it was stored in the House of God in Jerusalem. According to Herodotus, Frankincense was offered at the feast of Bel in Babylon. It also became the only incense offered to the Greek gods. The Romans used it not only in religious ceremonies but also in their domestic life. It is still one of the main incenses burned in Christian churches.

THERAPEUTIC EFFECTS

Negative charging molecules (1), anti-catarrhal, anti-depressive, cicatrisant (helps the repair of cuts and small wounds), expectorant, immunostimulant (encourages the optimal functioning of the immune system).

INDICATIONS AND COMMON USES
Therapeutic value ★★★

PHYSICAL SPHERE
■ **Respiratory system:** very beneficial for the treatment of asthma, bronchitis.
■ **Immune system:** Frankincense is very good for strengthening our natural immunity.

PSYCHO-SPIRITUAL SPHERE
Frankincense can be used for nervous depression, strength, protection,

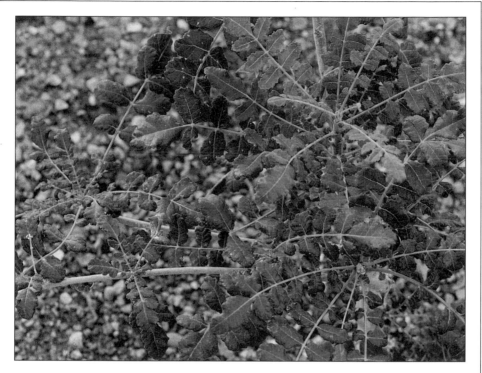

CHEMICAL CONSTITUENTS OF ESSENTIAL OIL

TERPENES:

■ Monoterpenes (40%): (alpha) pinene, limonene
■ Sesquiterpenes: (alpha) gurjurene, (alpha) guaiene

ALCOHOLS:

■ Monoterpenic alcohols: borneol, transpinocarveol, farnesol
■ Bi-functional compounds: alcohol-ketone: olibanol, alcohol-oxide: incensol oxide

enlightenment and reducing tension. It is calming, awakening the higher self and spiritual awareness. In meditation it opens and works through the brow and crown chakras.

⬛ BLENDS WELL WITH

Bergamot, Cypress, Myrrh, Sandalwood, Orange, Pine, Lemon, Ylang Ylang, Patchouli.

SAFETY PRECAUTIONS

None if used at the correct dosages.

CANAGA ODORATA FORMA GENUINA

Ylang Ylang

Ylang Ylang belongs to the *Anonanceae* family. The essential oil of Ylang Ylang is produced in Madagascar, Reunion, Commores, Sumatra, and the Philippines.

ESSENTIAL OIL

This is obtained by hydro-distillation from the flowers. It is a Top Note oil (according to other authors,

Middle Note) with a moist, grounding temperament and a very sweet, feminine, heady floral scent, and a yellow color.

THE PLANT

Ylang Ylang means "flower of flowers" in Malay. However, it is also accorded a Philippino derivation from *alang ilang*, flowers that flutter in the

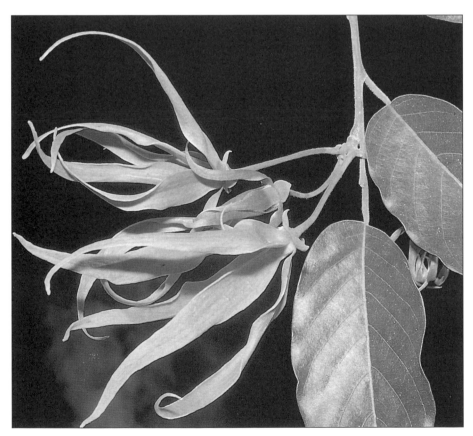

wind. The trees require a great deal of care in the autumn to be able to reach their usual heights of around 65 feet. The Ylang Ylang tree has long hanging stems with about 18 leaves on each. The wonderful beautiful flowers are narrow, downy, pale yellow, almost white in color, with long, tongue-shaped and shiny leaves. The trees need a lot of care: they must be trimmed every two months and the hand harvest of the flowers takes place yearly during the fall.

THERAPEUTIC EFFECTS

Negative charging molecules (1), anti-spasmodic, anti-depressant, aphrodisiac ★★, antiseptic, balancing ★★★, calming, hypotensor, sedative, soothing.

INDICATIONS AND COMMON USES
Therapeutic value ★★★

PHYSICAL CONDITIONS
■ **Circulation:** Ylang Ylang reduces high blood pressure, and is enhanced by its calming and soothing quality which gives very good results by eliminating tension and anxiety. Good for palpitations and tachycardia.
■ **Skin:** Ylang Ylang is a good skin-balancing oil for oily skin.

PSYCHO-SPIRITUAL
This oil is beneficial for hyperpnea

CHEMICAL CONSTITUENTS OF ESSENTIAL OIL

TERPENES:
■ Sesquiterpenes: (alpha) farnesene
ALCOHOLS:
■ Monoterpenic and aromatic alcohols: linalol (55%), benzylic alcohol
■ Sesquiterpenic alcohols: farnesol
ESTERS:
■ Geranyl acetate, benzyl acetate, benzyl benzoate
ETHERS:
■ Phenol-Methyl-Ether: P-cresol Methyl Ether

(increase in the number of breaths taken each minute), depression, frigidity, impotence, insomnia (sleeplessness), and tension.

BLENDS WELL WITH

Sandalwood, Lavender, Lemon, Myrrh, Benzoin, Bergamot, Patchouli, Cedarwood.

SAFETY PRECAUTIONS

Ylang Ylang, used sensibly, has no known side effects.

BITTER ORANGE

The Bitter Orange tree grows to a height of 32 feet and has dark green shiny, oval leaves, with white flowers and fleshy petals. The Bitter Orange fruits, known as Seville oranges, are small when compared with sweet oranges.

The Bitter Orange was first introduced to Europe from Southeast Asia in the tenth and eleventh centuries by the Arabs, and later taken to the Americas by the Spanish conquistadors. It produces three diverse essential oils: Neroli, Orange, and Petitgrain.

CITRUS AURANTIUM SSP AMARA

Neroli

Neroli belongs to the *Rutaceae* family. The essential oil of Neroli is produced in France, Italy, Morocco, and Tunisia.

ESSENTIAL OIL

The essential oil is produced by steam distillation of the petals of the fresh unopened flowers.

Neroli is a Middle to Top Note oil with a refreshing, cooling and moisture-balancing temperament, a fresh, spicy, bitter, floral scent, and a pale yellow color.

THE PLANT

In the later half of the sixteenth century, the Italian naturalist della Porta

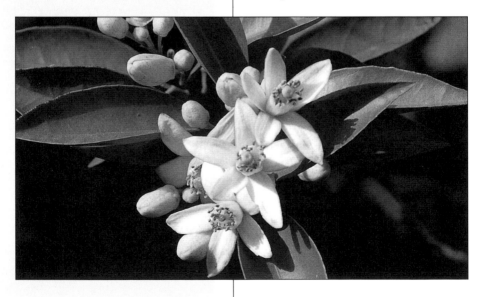

mentions the distilled oil of orange blossoms. In the seventeenth century this oil was renamed Neroli in honor of the Italian princess Anna Maria de la Tremoille, who had the title of Princess of Neroli.

THERAPEUTIC EFFECTS

Positive charging molecules (2), anti-infectious: anti-bacterial (makes the body tissues' environment inhospitable for pathogenic bacteria), anti-depressive (combats depression), hypotensive (lowers high blood pressure), digestive tonic, tonic for the liver and pancreas, tonic for the nervous system, phlebotonic (has a tonic effect on the walls of veins).

INDICATIONS AND COMMON USES:
Therapeutic value ★★★

PHYSICAL SPHERE
■ **Respiratory system:** is very good in a synergistic blend for bronchitis, pleurisy.
■ **Digestive system:** helps in enterocolitis, liver and pancreatic malfunctioning.
■ **Circulatory system:** this oil contributes to the treatment of hemorrhoids (piles), hypertension (high blood pressure), varicose veins.

PSYCHO-SPIRITUAL SPHERE
This oil is beneficial for those suffering from fatigue, tension, depression, and worry. In meditation it opens and balances the solar plexus chakra.

CHEMICAL CONSTITUENTS OF ESSENTIAL OIL

TERPENES:
■ Monoterpenes (35%): (alpha) pinene, (beta) pinene (17%), limonene

ALCOHOLS:
■ Aromatic alcohols: phenyl-ethylic alcohol, benzilic alcohol
■ Monoterpenic alcohols (40%): linalol 30–32%, (alpha) terpineol, geraniol, nerol (1.5%).
■ Sesquiterpenic alcohols (6%): trans nerolidol, farnesol I and II

ESTERS:
■ Terpenic esters: linalyl acetate, neryl acetate, geranyl acetate

ALDEHYDES:
■ 2,5 di-methyl—2—vinyl—hex 4 enal, decanal, benzaldehyde

KETONES:
■ Jasmone

AZOATED (N) COMPOUNDS:
■ Methyl anthranilate (0.6%), indole (0.1%)

BLENDS WELL WITH

Petitgrain, Orange, all other citrus oils, True Lavender, Rose, Rosewood, Sandalwood.

SAFETY PRECAUTIONS

None described.

CITRUS AURANTIUM SSP AMARA *continued*

PETITGRAIN (ORANGE)
Citrus aurantium ssp amara

 ### ESSENTIAL OIL

Petitgrain belongs to the *Rutaceae* family. It is extracted by steam distillation from the leaves, twigs and small, green buds of the Bitter Orange tree in France, Paraguay, Italy, Morocco, Brazil, and the United States.

Petitgrain is a Middle to Base Note oil with a warming and balancing temperament, a light, gentle, sweet yet lively and fruity scent, and a light yellow color.

 ### THE PLANT

The name is derived from the

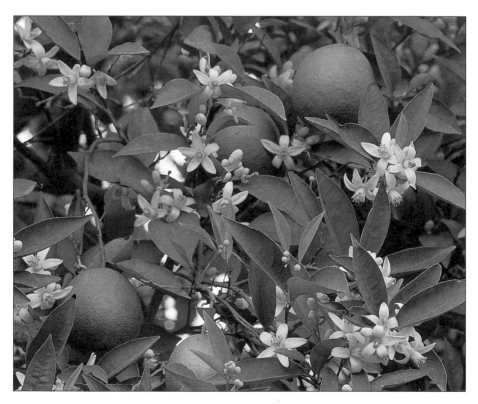

little green buds, *petit grains*, which are part of the distillation material.

THERAPEUTIC EFFECTS

Negative charging molecules (1), antiseptic, anti-bacterial ★, anti-inflammatory, major anti-spasmodic (relieves cramps), nervous rebalancer.

INDICATIONS AND COMMON USES
Therapeutic value ★ ★ ★

PHYSICAL SPHERE
■ **Digestive system:** good for benign chronic hepatitis.
■ **Skin:** good in formulations for acne.
■ **Nervous system:** helpful for neurovegetative dystonia, neuritis, inflammation of the peripheral nerve endings.
■ **Respiratory system:** a helpful ingredient of synergistic blends for respiratory infections.
■ **Female reproductive system:** this oil is a beneficial integral part of blends for premenstrual syndrome, menopausal stress, and tension.

PSYCHO-SPIRITUAL SPHERE
A very good oil for those in need of joy, or who are suffering from insomnia due to

CHEMICAL CONSTITUENTS OF ESSENTIAL OIL

TERPENES:
■ Monoterpenes (10%): myrcene, cis and trans ocimenes, paracimene

ALCOHOLS:
■ Monoterpenic alcohols (30–40%): linalol, terpineol, nerol, terpineol 4

ESTERS:
■ (50–75%): linalyl acetate, terpenyl acetate, neryl acetate, geranyl acetate

COMPOUNDS:
■ Di methyl anthranilate low %

an over-active mind or worry, Petitgrain also helps to overcome emotional shocks. In meditation it opens and balances the heart and throat chakras.

BLENDS WELL WITH

Eucalyptus Citriodoria, Bergamot, Cypress, Orange, Lemon, Patchouli, Ylang Ylang.

SAFETY PRECAUTIONS

None at therapeutic dosages.

CITRUS AURANTIUM SSP AMARA *continued*

ORANGE

Citrus aurantium ssp amara

ESSENTIAL OIL

Orange belongs to the *Rutaceae* family. The essential oil of Orange is produced in Israel, France, Italy, Spain, Morocco, Tunisia, and the United States.

This essential oil is obtained by cold expression from the rind of the bitter Orange fruit. It is a Top Note oil with a refreshing yet warming temperament, a light, gentle, sweet yet lively and

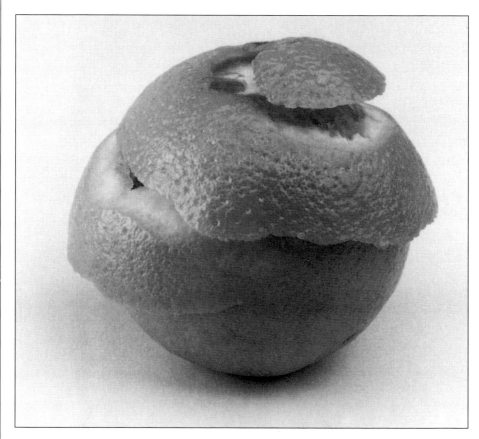

CHEMICAL CONSTITUENTS OF ESSENTIAL OIL

Volatile Fraction:

TERPENES:

■ Monoterpenes (90–92%): limonene (90%), terpinolene

ALCOHOLS:

■ Monoterpenic alcohols (0.4–3%): linalol, (alpha) terpineol, citronelol, nerol, geraniol

ESTERS:

■ (2%): geranyl acetate, neryl acetate, citronellyl acetate, linalyl acetate

ALDEHYDES:

■ (0.8–7%): nonalal, decanal, undecanal,

dodecanal, geranial, neral, citronelal

CUMARINES AND FUROCUMARINES:

■ Auraptene, auraptenol, bergaptene, bergaptol, soparone, citroptene

Non volatile fraction:

FLAVONOIDS:

■ Triterpenoid (beta) carotenes, steroids, fatty acids

COUMARINES AND FUROCOUMARINES

■ Substitutes.

---

fruity scent, and a dark yellow to light orange color.

THERAPEUTIC EFFECTS

Negative charging molecules (1), calming, sedative, anti-inflammatory, tonic, mild anti-coagulant.

INDICATIONS AND COMMON USES

Therapeutic value ★★

PHYSICAL SPHERE

■ **Circulatory system:** for general circulation disorders.

■ **Digestive system:** beneficial for dyspepsia, flatulence, gastric colic.

PSYCHO-SPIRITUAL SPHERE

Used for treating anxiety, tension, vertigo. In meditation it balances the root chakra and opens the solar plexus chakra.

BLENDS WELL WITH

Bergamot, Cinnamon leaves, Lemon, Ginger, Marjoram, Neroli, Petitgrain, Sandalwood and Ylang Ylang.

SAFETY PRECAUTIONS

Photosensitizing action can cause sunburn if used before exposure to sun.

CITRUS AURANTIUM SSP BERGAMIA

Bergamot

Bergamot belongs to the *Rutaceae* family. Bergamot trees grow in Italy (Reggio di Calabria), Corsica, the Ivory Coast, Tunisia, and Algeria.

ESSENTIAL OIL

The essential oil of Bergamot is obtained from the rind of the unripe, very bitter and sour Bergamot fruit, a small variety of citrus fruit, and is extracted by cold expression and centrifugation. The oil thus gained is highly esteemed by the perfume industry and is an ingredient of commercial Eau de Cologne formulations and Earl Grey tea.

Bergamot is a Top Note oil with a warming and balancing temperament, a light, gentle, sweet yet lively and fruity scent which is equally loved by both sexes. It is a light green color.

THE PLANT

The bergamot tree grows up to 16 feet in height, has dark green, oval leaves, star-shaped flowers, and small pear-shaped green fruits which ripen to a yellow color and are similar in appearance to quinces.

The Bergamot tree is thought to be originally from Asia, possibly New Guinea, India, or Burma. According to Italian

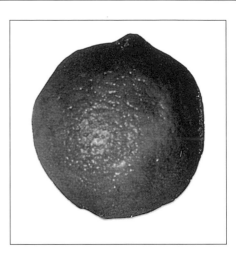

folklore, the name originates from the city of Bergamo in Lombardy, southern Italy. However, further research leads us to *Beg br m dn*, which means Prince of Burma; it is said that later the Turkish name was corrupted to Bergamot. The fruit has been used locally for medicinal purposes since the sixteenth century. Prior to the end of the seventeenth century there is no mention of this tree. In the later part of 1677 we can find an entry in the German *pharmacopea*. It is since this period that we are able to trace a mention of Bergamot in the recipes of various fragrant waters, or Eau de Cologne. J.M. Farina, the creator of the original Eau de Cologne recipe, was inspired by the sister of the convent of Santa Maria Novella in Florence. Professor Paolo Rovesti has conducted extensive research into the use of Bergamot in psychotherapy for patients suffering from fears and phobias and in treatments for weight loss and alcoholism.

THERAPEUTIC EFFECTS

Negative charging molecules (1), analgesic, anti-depressant, antiseptic, anti-spasmodic, digestive, expectorant, healing of the skin, stimulant, relaxing, revitalizing, uplifting.

INDICATIONS AND COMMON USES

Therapeutic value: ★★★

PHYSICAL SPHERE

■ **Skin:** acne, eczema.

■ **Digestive system:** Bergamot regulates and balances the appetite and is particularly useful for eating disorders such as anorexia and bulimia nervosa. Bergamot is also beneficial for the treatment of nausea and vomiting.

■ **Respiratory system:** Bergamot is beneficial for bronchitis, catarrh, coughs, colds, cold sores.

■ **Urinary system:** in cases of cystitis, urethritis.

■ **Female reproductive system:** Bergamot is helpful in vulvar and vaginal pruritus (itchiness), leucorrhoea (vaginal discharges), vaginitis (vaginal inflammations and infections), thrush (vaginal discharge due to *Candida albicans*, a fungus).

PSYCHO-SPIRITUAL SPHERE

It is in the realm of emotions that Bergamot is at its best, such as in the treatment of depression and nervous tension; in

CHEMICAL CONSTITUENTS OF ESSENTIAL OIL

TERPENES:

■ Monoterpenes: (alpha) pinene, camphene, limonene

ALCOHOLS

■ Aromatic Alcohols: Di-hydrocuninic alcohol, Monoterpenic alcohols: linalol, nerol, geraniol, terpineol

ALDEHYDES:

■ citrals

ESTERS:

■ linalyl acetate 29%

FUROCUMARINS:

■ bergamotine, bergaptene, bergaptole, auraptenole, angelicine, limetine, 5–geranoxy–7–metoxy coumarine

meditation, Bergamot opens with the heart chakra and the solar plexus chakra.

BLENDS WELL WITH

Frankincense, Geranium, Mandarin, Melissa, Myrtle, Neroli, Palmarosa, Sandalwood, Vetiver and Ylang Ylang.

SAFETY PRECAUTIONS

Bergamot can be a skin irritant in high concentrations and can also produce a very uneven tan or cause a burn if used up to 12 hours before exposure to strong sunshine due to its photosensitizing action.

CITRUS LIMONUM
Lemon

This belongs to the *Rutaceae* family. The Lemon tree grows around the Mediterranean, in Florida, California, Argentina, and Brazil.

ESSENTIAL OIL

The essential oil is obtained from the rind of fresh Lemons by cold expression and centrifugation. It is a Top Note oil with a warming and balancing temperament, a light, lively and fruity scent, and a pale yellow color with a greenish tinge.

THE PLANT

The Lemon tree reaches 10–20 feet in height, with pale to dark green leaves, with oil-rich protuberances in the branches. The flowers are mainly white although sometimes they may be pink.

THERAPEUTIC EFFECTS

Positive charging molecules (2), anti-acid, anti-infectious: anti-bacterial, anti-viral, anti-helmintic, anti-neuralgic, anti-pruritic, antiseptic, spores, astringent,

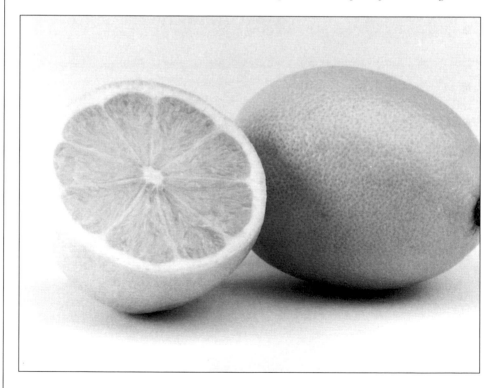

calming ★★, cicatrisant, diuretic, febrifugue (lowers fevers), hemostatic (helps to control bleeding), hepatic, hypotensive (lowers blood pressure), stimulant, tonic.

INDICATIONS AND COMMON USES
Therapeutic value ★★

Note: Lemon is an air antiseptic.

PHYSICAL SPHERE
■ **Digestive system:** essential oil of Lemon is beneficial in blends for indigestion.

■ **Skin:** Lemon is good in blends for cold sores and other types of herpes.

■ **Circulation:** beneficial in blends for hypertension, varicose veins, venous malfunctioning.

■ **Urinary system:** good in blends for edema, renal colics.

■ **Respiratory system:** beneficial in blends for many respiratory infections.

■ **Joints and muscles:** essential oil of Lemon is beneficial in blends for rheumatism.

PSYCHO-SPIRITUAL SPHERE
Essential oil of Lemon is beneficial in blends for anxiety, concentration, and insomnia. It relieves stress and tension. In meditation it balances all chakras, and opens the heart and throat chakra.

CHEMICAL CONSTITUENTS OF ESSENTIAL OIL

TERPENES:
■ Monoterpenes: limonene, terpinene (alpha), terpinene (gamma), phellandrene (alpha), phelandrene (beta), terpinolene

SESQUITERPENES:
■ Bisabolene (alpha)

ALCOHOLS:
■ Aliphatic: hexanol, octanol, nonanol, decanol, 3 hexenelol, heptanol

ALDEHYDES
■ Hexanol, heptanal, octanal, nonanal, geranial

CUMARINS AND FUROCUMARINS
■ Scopoletine, umbcliferone, bergaptine, bergaptole, bergaptene, citropiene, geranoxipsoralene (delta), 5–geranoxi–8–metoxi psoralene
■ Non-volatile constituents 2% flavonoids, carotenoids, steriods, cumarins

BLENDS WELL WITH
Bergamot, Cypress, Frankincense, Ginger, Orange, Petitgrain, Sandalwood, Rosewood.

SAFETY PRECAUTIONS
Essential oil of Lemon may give photosensitivity.

COMMIPHORA MOLMOL, COMMYPHORA MYRRHA

Myrrh

Myrrh belongs to the *Burseraceae* family. It grows in Africa, mainly Somalia, Yemen and Ethiopia, and when tapped exudes a gum which solidifies when in contact with the air.

ESSENTIAL OIL

The essential oil is obtained by steam distillation from the resinoid. It is a Base Note oil with a warming temperament, a smoky, bitter, slightly musty scent and a dark, reddish-brown color.

THE PLANT

The bushes yielding the resin do not grow over nine feet. They are sturdy with lots of branches which stand out at right angles ending in a sharp spine and scanty, small, uneven leaves. There are ducts in the bark, and the tissue between them breaks down forming large cavities which, with the remaining ducts, become filled with a granular secretion which freely discharges when the bark is wounded. It flows as a pale yellow liquid which hardens to a reddish-brown mass. It is found as tears of varying sizes, the average being the size of a small nut.

Myrrh was well known to the ancient Egyptians, part of the well-known Kyphy. Moses took it with him when the

CHEMICAL CONSTITUENTS OF ESSENTIAL OIL

HYDROCARBONS:
- Isopropenyl furane (4.5%)

TERPENES:
- Sesquiterpenes: elemene, copaene, furanic sesquiterpenes: curzerene

KETONES:
- Methyl isobutyl ketone

ALDEHYDES:
- Methyl 1, 2 butenal

Israelites left Egypt, and it was one of the gifts to Jesus from the Magi, as it was considered very precious. Valerius Cordius, Gerard and Gestner described how to prepare ointments with the resin which were used in the treatment of cuts and wounds.

THERAPEUTIC EFFECTS

Negative charging molecules (1), anti-viral ★★★, antiseptic, astringent, anti-inflammatory, fungicide, expectorant, stimulating, sedative, thyroid hormone regulator, tonic.

INDICATIONS AND COMMON USES
Therapeutic value ★★★

PHYSICAL SPHERE

■ **Female reproductive system:** Myrrh is beneficial in synergistic formulations for amenorrhea (lack of periods).

■ **Respiratory system:** beneficial for catarrh and coughs.

■ **Digestive system:** of benefit for diarrhea, dyspepsia, flatulence, gingivitis (gums), loss of appetite, sequels of viral hepatitis.

■ **Endocrine glands:** Myrrh is good in the synergistic formulation for hyperthyroidism.

■ **Skin and mucus membranes:** Myrrh is beneficial in synergistic formulation for pyorrhea (pus in gums), mouth and skin ulcers, athlete's foot, wounds.

PSYCHO-SPIRITUAL SPHERE

Myrrh gives strength and courage, it quickens awareness of the spiritual reality. In meditation it opens and balances all chakras.

 ## BLENDS WELL WITH

Bergamot, Frankincense, Geranium, Sandalwood, Rose, Rosewood, Ylang Ylang.

SAFETY PRECAUTIONS

None if used sensibly.

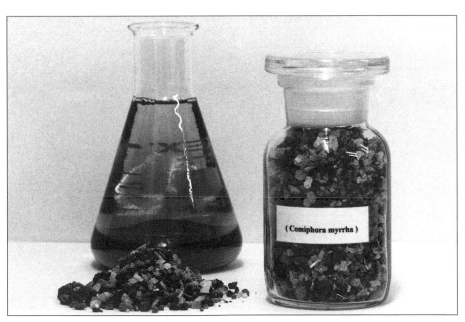

(Comiphora myrrha)

CUPRESSUS SEMPERVIRENS

Cypress

Cypress belongs to the *Cupresaceae* family. The essential oil of Cypress is produced in France and Spain.

ESSENTIAL OIL

This is extracted by steam distillation from the needles and twigs of the Cypress tree. The essential oil of Cypress is a Middle Note oil with a cooling temperament and a fresh, woody, balsamic scent, and greenish-yellow color.

THE PLANT

The Cypress is a tall and slender evergreen conifer, which grows up to 80–96 feet tall and has a reddish-yellow colored bark.

The medicinal use of Cypress can be traced back to the ancient Egyptians. The Greeks dedicated the tree to Hades, god of the underworld, and for them it symbolized everlasting life; the ancient physician Galen recommended its use for internal hemorrhoids and bleeding. It was also recommended during this period for menstrual disorders.

THERAPEUTIC EFFECTS

Positive charging molecules (2), antiseptic, astringent, bronchial anti-spasmodic, circulatory tonic, diuretic, enterotonic, hepatic, venous decongestant, lymphatic decongestant, neurotonic.

INDICATIONS AND COMMON USES
Therapeutic value ★★★

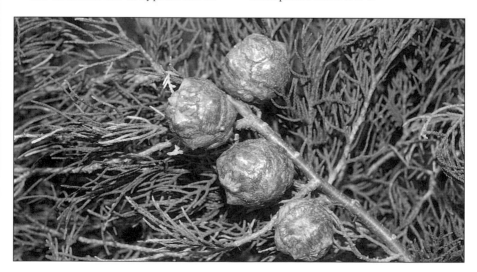

PHYSICAL SPHERE

■ **Respiratory system:** Cypress is helpful for asthma, bronchitic coughs and whooping cough.

■ **Immune system:** Cypress is very good in hay fever caused by tree pollen.

■ **Circulatory system:** the essential oil of Cypress is beneficial for bleeding gums, hemorrhage, hemorrhoids, edema (swelling) of the lower limbs, and varicose veins.

■ **Genito-urinary system:** Cypress helps incontinence sufferers and also prostatic adenomas (benign growths).

■ **Female reproductive system:** Cypress is one of the oils of choice in dysmenorrhea (painful periods).

■ **Skin:** in skincare, oil of Cypress is used because of its astringent properties. It is very good for oily skin.

PSYCHO-SPIRITUAL SPHERE

Cypress provides solace in times of bereavement; it is calming and soothing in times of transition and when difficult changes are required. Cypress is ideal where completion, clearing, synthesis, grounding or consolidation are required; it is beneficial in asthenia (extreme tiredness and despondency) and tension. It is good for meditation and solace, and helps people to come to terms with bereavement. It is good for balancing the root and solar plexus chakras, a valuable

CHEMICAL CONSTITUENTS OF ESSENTIAL OIL

TERPENES:
■ Monoterpenes: (alpha) pinene, (delta) 3 carene
■ Sesquiterpenes: (alpha) cimene, (delta) cadimene

ALCOHOLS:
■ Sesquiterpenols: cedrol, labdanic di-terpenols: manol, sempervirol

ACIDS:
■ Diterpenic acids: neocupresic acid

oil for the heart chakra, and the whole green area covering the heart and lungs. In those wishing to connect with the higher or inner self during meditation it aids the meeting of logic and intuition leading to perfection and attainment.

BLENDS WELL WITH

 Bergamot, Roman Chamomile, Clary Sage, Cedarwood, Geranium, Hyssop, Juniper, Lavender, Lemon, Lemongrass, Mandarin, Pine, Spruce, Rock Rose, Rosemary, Thyme Linalol.

SAFETY PRECAUTIONS

None at recommended dosages.

EUCALYPTUS CITRIODORA

Eucalyptus Citriodora

This belongs to the *Myrtaceae* family. The essential oil of Eucalyptus Citriodora is produced in Australia, North America, and South America.

ESSENTIAL OIL

The essential oil is obtained by steam distillation from the leaves of the Eucalyptus Citriodora. It is a Top Note oil

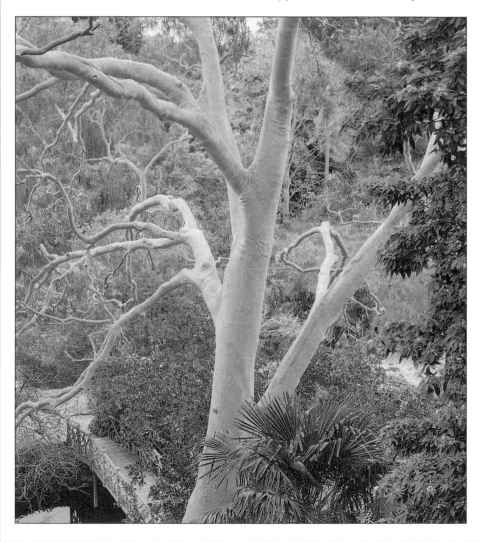

with a cooling yet warming temperament. It has a light, fresh, citrusy sweet yet lively scent, and a clear to light yellow color.

THE PLANT

This species of Eucalyptus has fluffy white flowers.

THERAPEUTIC EFFECTS

Major negative charging oil (1), anti-inflammatory, anti-rheumatic, a good analgesic, antiseptic, anti-diabetic (certain types of diabetes), anti-spasmodic (minor use), calming, hypotensor, sedative.

INDICATIONS AND COMMON USES

Therapeutic value ★★★

PHYSICAL SPHERE

■ **Joints:** Eucalyptus Citriodora is beneficial for the treatment of arthritis and rheumatism.

■ **Urinary system:** good for cystitis (bladder infections).

■ **Circulation:** it is very useful in a formulation for hypertension (high blood pressure).

■ **For viral infections of the nerve endings:** Eucalyptus Citriodora is good for shingles.

■ **Female reproductive system:** Eucalyptus Citriodora is good for vaginitis, inflammations of the vaginal canal with or without infections.

CHEMICAL CONSTITUENTS OF ESSENTIAL OIL

ALCOHOLS:
■ Monoterpenic alcohols: citronelol, trans pino carveol, geraniol, cis and trans p menthane 3–8 diols

ESTERS:
■ Monoterpenic esters: citronelil acetate, citronelil butirate, citronelil citronelate

ALDEHYDES:
■ Monoterpenic aldehydes: citronelal (40–80%)

PSYCHO-SPIRITUAL SPHERE

In meditation, the essential oil of Eucalyptus Citriodora opens the heart and throat chakras, lightens a heavy heart and induces breathing.

BLENDS WELL WITH

Bergamot, Cypress, Lemon, Orange, other Eucalypti, Sandalwood, Ylang Ylang.

SAFETY PRECAUTIONS

A safe oil if used correctly following established guidelines.

EUCALYPTUS GLOBULUS

Eucalyptus Globulus

Eucalyptus Globulus belongs to the *Myrtaceae* family. It is indigenous to Australia, and for centuries has also grown in Ecuador and Bolivia and is being cultivated in China.

ESSENTIAL OIL

The essential oil is obtained by steam distillation from the leaves of the Eucalyptus tree. It is a Top Note oil with a warming and balancing temperament, a herby, camphorous, lively and medicinal scent, and a dark yellow color.

THE PLANT

Eucalyptus Globulus is a tall tree which can grow up to 328 feet, with a smooth white bark, and slender, sickle-shaped long silvery leaves, and large fluffy white flowers.

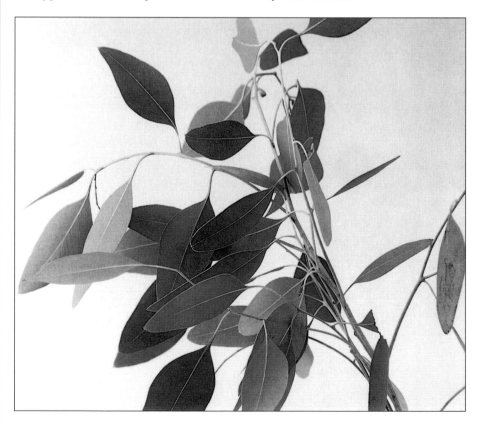

THERAPEUTIC EFFECTS

Positive charging molecules (2), analgesic (pain killer), antiseptic, anti-spasmodic, anti-rheumatic, anti-catarrhal, bactericidal, deodorant, diuretic (helps fluid retention), expectorant (helps to eliminate mucus from the lungs), urinary antiseptic.

INDICATIONS AND COMMON USES

Therapeutic value ★★★

PHYSICAL SPHERE

- **General:** fevers, insect repellent.
- **Muscles and joints:** good for the treatment of muscular aches and pains, rheumatic pains.
- **Respiratory system:** may be used for asthma under medical supervision, bronchitis, coughs, sinusitis, throat infections by using inhalations.
- **For viral infections:** helps in flu, measles, chickenpox and other childhood diseases.
- **Skin:** for some skin ulcers and wounds because of its antiseptic properties.

PSYCHO-SPIRITUAL SPHERE

This oil is good for migraine sufferers. It alleviates mental exhaustion and feelings of loneliness. In meditation it opens and balances the heart and throat chakras.

Note: a steam inhalation with Eucalyptus is effective for coughs and colds not only

CHEMICAL CONSTITUENTS OF ESSENTIAL OIL

TERPENES:
- Monoterpenes: (alpha) pinene, (beta) pinene
- Sesquiterpenes: aromadendrene, allo aromadendrene, delta guaiazulene

ALCOHOLS:
- Aliphatic and monoterpenic alcohols: transpinocarveol
- Sesquiterpenic alcohols or sesquiterpenols: globulol ledol

KETONES:
- Monoterpenones: (–) pinocarvone, carvone

OXYDES:
- Terpenic oxydes: 1–8 cineole

ALDEHYDES:
- Butiraldehyde, valer-aldehyde, capro-aldehyde

because it is a decongestant but also because of its anti-viral action.

BLENDS WELL WITH

Bergamot, Roman Chamomile, True Lavender, Frankincense, Neroli, Ginger, Lemon.

SAFETY PRECAUTIONS

Not to be used in infants or young children.

LAVANDULA OFFICINALIS, ANGUSTIFOLIA, VERA

Lavender (fine)

This belongs to the family of the *Labiatae*, also known as *Lamiaceae*. True Lavender grows mainly in Bulgaria, China, Croatia, England, France, Russia, and Tasmania.

ESSENTIAL OIL

The essential oil is obtained by steam distillation from the flowering tops. It is a Top to Middle Note oil with a soothing, comforting temperament, a flowery, fresh scent reminiscent of old linen, and a clear color.

THE PLANT

The plant is an evergreen woody shrub which grows up to 39 inches in height. It has pale green, linear leaves and beautiful violet-blue flowers. It is versatile but it grows best on a high, dry, sunny plateau where it appreciates the wind and likes the minerals in the soil. High-altitude *angustifolia*, whether cultivated or wild, is likely to produce more esters; plants growing in lowland areas will be of less value therapeutically. High-altitude Lavender harnesses natural power and energy which gives it an uplifting quality and enhances its therapeutic value. Some Lavender is not cultivated, but true harvesting of the wild plant is still a tradition and is of a skillful nature as the wild plant carries fewer flowers and must be picked at exactly the right time to produce the essential oil at its peak.

THERAPEUTIC EFFECTS

Negative charging molecules (1), anti-catarrhal, analgesic, antiseptic, anti-infectious, anti-bacterial, anti-viral, anti-fungal, expectorant, cardiotonic, cytophylactic, general tonic, wound healing.

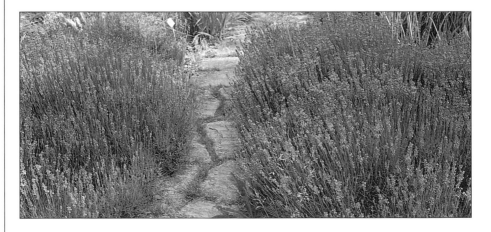

INDICATIONS AND COMMON USES
Therapeutic value ★★★★

PHYSICAL SPHERE
■ **Respiratory tract:** beneficial in the treatment of rhynitis (hay fever), viral tracheo bronchitis, otitis (ear infections), loose dry cough, tonsillitis.

■ **Digestive system:** True Lavender is beneficial for viral enterocolitis.

■ **Joints and muscles:** good for rheumatism, rheumatoid arthritis.

■ **Peripheral nerves:** for neuritis, neuralgia.

■ **Skin:** good for acne, dry eczema, severe burns ★★★.

PSYCHO-SPIRITUAL SPHERE
True Lavender is very good for those suffering from asthenia (extreme tiredness and despondency), depression, insomnia, nervous tension, stress due to parasympathetic nervous overload.

BLENDS WELL WITH
Bergamot, Roman Chamomile, German Chamomile, other Lavenders, Mandarin, Neroli, Orange, Jasmine, Melissa, Rosemary, Rosewood, Sandalwood.

SAFETY PRECAUTIONS
None at recommended dosages and if used correctly.

CHEMICAL CONSTITUENTS OF ESSENTIAL OIL

TERPENES:
■ Monoterpenes: high percentages of (alpha) pinene, (beta) pinene, camphene, carene, cis and trans ocimenes, allocimene, limonene
■ Sesquiterpenes: (beta) caryophyllene, (beta) farnesene

ALCOHOLS:
■ Monoterpenic alcohols: linalol, terpinene 1 ol 4, terpineol, borneol, geraniol, lavandulol

ALDEHYDES:
■ Trans 2 hexanal (0.4%), cuminal (0.43%), benzaldehyde (0.2%), neral, geranial (0.48%), myrtenal (0.17%)

KETONES:
■ Non terpenic and terpenic octanone 1.3%, para methyl aceto phenone, camphone
■ Sesquiterpenones: mono and bi cycllic 2%

OXYDES (35%):
■ 1,8 cineole, eucalyptole (25–38%), caryophyllene oxide, linalol oxides

ESTERS:
■ Linalyl acetate, terpenyl acetate, geranyl acetate, lavandulyl acetate

LACTONES:
■ Less than 1% butanolids

CUMARINES (0.25%):
■ Cumarin 0.04%, herniarine, umbeliferone, santoline

LAVANDULA SPICA, LATIFOLIA

Lavender (spike)

This belongs to the family of the *Labiatae*, also known as *Lamiaceae*. Spike Lavender grows in France, Spain, and Tasmania.

ESSENTIAL OIL

The essential oil of Spike Lavender is obtained by steam distillation from the flowering tops. It is a Top Note oil with a warming and balancing temperament, a warm, slightly medicinal lively, camphorous scent, and clear color.

THERAPEUTIC EFFECTS

Negative charging molecules (1),

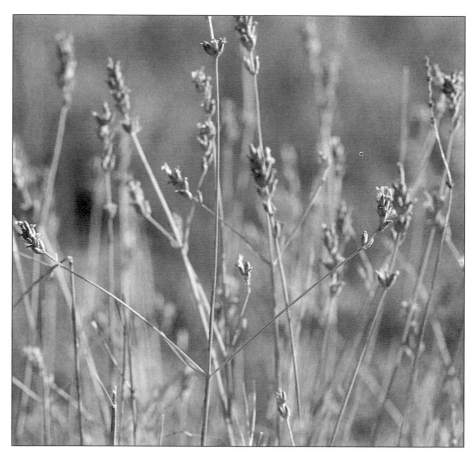

analgesic, antiseptic, microbicidal, anti-infectious: anti-bacterial H, anti-viral ★★★★, anti-fungal, expectorant, anti-catarrhal, cardiotonic, general tonic.

INDICATIONS AND COMMON USES
Therapeutic value ★★★

PHYSICAL SPHERE
■ **Respiratory tract:** Spike Lavender is beneficial in synergistic blends for rhynitis, viral tracheo bronchitis, otitis, loose dry cough, tonsillitis.

■ **Digestive system:** Spike Lavender is good in synergistic blends for viral enterocolitis.

■ **Joints and muscles:** in synergistic blends for rheumatism, rheumatoid arthritis.

■ **Peripheral nerves:** beneficial in synergistic blends for neuritis and neuralgia.

■ **Skin:** it is beneficial in synergistic blends for acne, dry eczema, severe burns.

PSYCHO-SPIRITUAL SPHERE
Spike Lavender is beneficial in synergistic blends for over-tiredness, anxiety and tension.

BLENDS WELL WITH
Eucalyptus Globulus, Roman Chamomile, other Lavenders, Rosewood, Sandalwood, Lemon, Ginger.

CHEMICAL CONSTITUENTS OF ESSENTIAL OILS

ALCOHOLS:
■ Monoterpenic alcohols: (alpha) terpineol

TERPENES:
■ Monoterpenes high percentages: (alpha) pinene, (beta) pinene
■ Sesquiterpenes: (beta) caryophyllene

KETONES:
■ (less than 15%): camphone (6–16%), carvone (0.1–0.5%)

OXYDES:
■ (35%): 1,8 cineole, eucalyptole (25–38%), caryophyllene oxide, cis and trans linalol oxides (tr 2.5 and cis 0.1–1.5%)

ESTERS:
■ (less than 2%): linalyl acetate (0.1–12.2%)

CUMARINES:
■ (0.2%): coumarine, herniarine

SAFETY PRECAUTIONS

None at recommended dosages.

LEPTOSPERMIUM SCOPARIUM

Manuka

Essential oil of Manuka belongs to the *Myrtaceae* family. Manuka is a native of New Zealand.

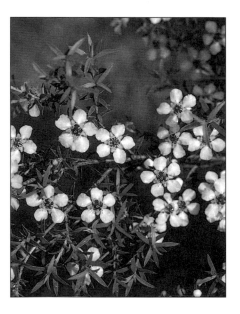 ESSENTIAL OIL

The essential oil is obtained by steam distillation of the leaves and twigs. It is a Top Note oil with a warming temperament, a fragrant, medicinal scent similar to that of tincture of benzoin, and a clear yellow-brown color. Manuka has been known for a long time in New Zealand. The marketing of the oil is currently being subsidized by the New Zealand government and numerous scientific studies regarding the anti-infectious value of the oil can be obtained from them.

THE PLANT

It is a small tree with red wood, dark green, pointed, sickle-shaped leaves characteristic of the *Myrtaceae*, and small red flowers in clusters.

In traditional Maori society, all knowledge of medicinal plants was held by medicinal herbalists, known as "tonunga," and gradually this knowledge became known to the rest of the people. The older women of the tribe kept the knowledge alive and ensured that it was handed down from generation to generation.

The accounts of early European settlers describe treatments of conditions such as skin infections, external wounds, burns and sores with Manuka. Internally, an infusion of the inner bark was used as a sedative for an excited person or someone in pain. As a digestive tonic for the treatment of constipation, dysentery and diarrhea, pieces of the bark were boiled until the water darkened in color and the liquid was then drunk.

THERAPEUTIC EFFECTS

Negative charging molecules (1). This oil has been proven to have a broad spectrum anti-bacterial action (with good effect on gram positive and gram negative

CHEMICAL CONSTITUENTS OF ESSENTIAL OIL

ALCOHOLS:
■ Sesquiterpenic alcohols (10.3%): spatulenol 0.4%, cubenol 0.86%

TERPENES:
■ Monoterpenes: high percentages ((alpha) pinene (1.08%), (beta) pinene (0.14%), myrcene (0.21%), limonene (0.17%), para cimene (0.2%)
■ Sesquiterpenes (26.4%): ylangene 0.32%, cubebene (4.3%), selinene ((4.3%), copaene, gurjurene (1.06%), caryophyllene (2.47%), humulene (5.5%)

OXIDES:
■ Sesquiterpenic oxides: caryophyllene epoxide 0.23%, other oxides 4.21%

KETONES:
■ Flavesone 5.18%, iso leptospermone 4.47%, leptospermone 15.93%

bacteria), a good anti-viral and anti-fungal action; in some studies the anti-viral effect proved to be better than that of *Melaleuca alternifolia*, Tea Tree. Due to its constituents it is a good expectorant and anti-catarrhal, anti-inflammatory, anti-histaminic, and nasal decongestant. A circulatory tonic with its main effect on the venous return.

INDICATIONS AND COMMON USES
Therapeutic value ★ ★ ★

PHYSICAL SPHERE
■ **Respiratory system:** upper and lower respiratory tract infections: sinusitis, tonsillitis, acute bronchitis, asthma.
■ **Joints and muscular system:** Manuka's anti-inflammatory properties make it a very useful oil for the treatment of muscular and articular conditions such as osteoarthritis and rheumatoid arthritis.

PSYCHO-SPIRITUAL SPHERE
Manuka is a warming, invigorating oil for not only physical but also spiritual coldness, inability to see sense in life, lack of the sparkle to live. If used for meditation it balances the solar plexus and throat chakras.

 ### BLENDS WELL WITH
Bergamot, Roman Chamomile, Eucalyptus Citriodora, Eucalyptus Radiata, Coriander, Pine, Spruce, and some others.

SAFETY PRECAUTIONS

Unlike Tea Tree, which is frequently used undiluted on the surface of the skin, Manuka is a moderate skin irritant and may cause redness and soreness when applied undiluted to the surface of the skin.

MATRICARIA RECUTITA OR MATRICARIA CHAMOMILLA

Chamomile (German)

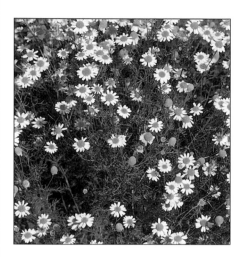

German Chamomile belongs to the *Compositae* family, also known as *Asteraceae* (the same family as the Roman Chamomile). It is also commonly known as Blue Chamomile, Wild Chamomile, Hungarian Chamomile, Ground Chamomile and Scented Mayweed.

German Chamomile is grown in Hungary, Slovakia, North America, Asia, and Australia and thus the essential oil is produced there.

ESSENTIAL OIL

This is extracted by steam distillation of the flowering tops. It has been estimated that 1100 pounds of flowering tops yield two pounds of essential oil. It is interesting to remember that it is no longer cultivated and distilled in Germany.

German Chamomile is a Base Note oil with a cooling and balancing temperament, a strong, herby-medicinal scent, and a deep blue color with a thick, viscous texture.

THE PLANT

The adult plant can reach eight to 20 inches in height. It is hairless with a short branching stem; the flower heads are about half an inch broad, with about 15 strap-shaped petals, numerous yellow, tubular, perfect florets, which do not have scales (a differentiating feature), and the receptacle is hollow.

In the Germanic tradition the longest day of the year was dedicated to the god Baldor. Legend tells us that at night Chamomile plants possessed magic qualities, and plants collected during the night had special healing powers. In the Middle Ages, Chamomile was spread on the stone floors of grand halls to dispose of bad smells. The Arab physician Avicenna prescribed Chamomile for female problems, hence the relation of the botanical name of Matricaria relating to "matrix" which is the Latin for womb. Chamomile was praised in the work of the German doctor J. Camerarius, the *Hortus Medicus et Philosophicus*, published in Frankfurt in 1588, in which he recommended Chamomile oil for colic.

During the sixteenth and seventeenth centuries, Chamomile was relegated to a secondary position in the garden, placed along garden paths so that it would release its aroma when walked on. Later it was recognized as the true plant healer; where Chamomile grew so did other healing plants.

THERAPEUTIC EFFECTS

Negative charging molecules. Analgesic, anti-allergic, and anti-inflammatory ★★, anti-spasmodic ★★, cicatrizing (helps to produce an even healing of cuts and wounds), decongestant, digestive tonic.

INDICATIONS AND COMMON USES
Therapeutic value ★★★

PHYSICAL SPHERE
■ **Female reproductive system:** amenorrhea and dysmenorrhea.
■ **Respiratory system:** bronchitis.
■ **Urinary system:** cystitis.
■ **Skin:** dermatitis, eczema, pruritus, psoriasis, and skin infections.
■ **Digestive system:** dyspepsia.

PSYCHO-SPIRITUAL SPHERE
Very beneficial for the overly sensitive, disagreeable and melancholic. In meditation, German Chamomile opens and balances the heart and throat chakras,

CHEMICAL CONSTITUENTS OF ESSENTIAL OIL

TERPENES:
■ Sesquiterpenes: chamazulene (less than 5%), dihydrochamazulenes I and II, bisabolenes, trans (farnesene)

ALCOHOLS:
■ Sesquiterpenols: (alpha) bisabolol, spathulenol and farnesol

SESQUITERPENIC OXYDES:
■ Bisabololoxyde A (23%), B (10%), C epoxy bisabolol

SESQUITERPENIC LACTONES

CUMARINES AND METOXICUMARINES:
■ Umbeliferone, herniarine

ETHERS:
■ Bi-ciclic polienic ether

it helps dissatisfaction, anger and self-centeredness, and helps all inflammations of the body and mind.

BLENDS WELL WITH

Benzoin, Bergamot, Roman Chamomile, Cypress, Frankincense, Mandarin, Neroli, Ravensara, Rosewood, Sandalwood, Spruce.

SAFETY PRECAUTIONS

None known at accepted conventional dosages.

MELALEUCA ALTERNIFOLIA

Tea Tree

Tea Tree belongs to the *Myrtaceae* family. It grows in Australia and Tasmania.

ESSENTIAL OIL

The essential oil of Tea Tree is obtained by steam distillation of the leaves and twigs. Tea tree is a Top Note oil with a temperament, a strong, fresh, medicinal scent, and pale yellow color.

THERAPEUTIC EFFECTS

Positive charging molecules (2), analgesic, anti-bacterial of wide spectrum: gram positive and gram negative, anti-fungal: candida, anti-viral, antiseptic and anti-inflammatory, antiasthenic, anti-diarrheic, cardiotonic, eubiotic (maintains friendly organisms alive), immuno-stimulant (increases IgA, and IgM), immunomodulant (maintains the healthy balance of the immune system), neurotonic, phlebotonic (tones the walls of surface veins), helps to protect the skin prior to radiotherapy (ask for the specialist's permission before utilizing any oils), venous decongestant.

INDICATIONS AND COMMON USES
Therapeutic value ★★★★

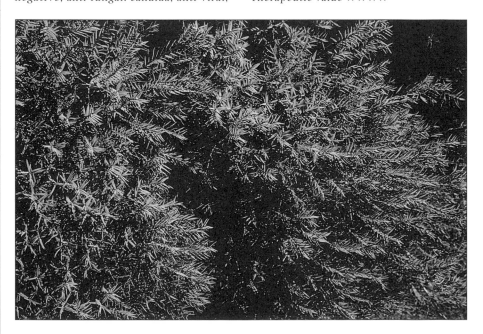

PHYSICAL SPHERE

■ **Skin:** Tea Tree helps to clear acne, athlete's foot, cold sores, spots (period spots).

■ **Respiratory system:** valuable for the treatment of infections such as bronchitis, colds, flu.

■ **Circulatory system:** Tea Tree invigorates and helps cardiac fatigue, hemorrhoids, varicose veins.

■ **Digestive system:** very useful in the treatment of mouth ulcers or stomatitis, gingivitis, enterocolitis.

■ **Genito-urinary system:** Tea Tree oil is very beneficial for bacterial genital infections.

■ **Immune system:** for strengthening the immune system in low resistance, shingles, surgical shock.

■ **Female reproductive system:** Tea Tree is very helpful in cases of thrush, vulvovaginitis.

PSYCHO-SPIRITUAL SPHERE

Tea Tree is very helpful to those suffering from deep grief, emotional pain, and anxiety. It also helps to calm down and balance an over-active mind when formulated with True Lavender and Roman Chamomile. In meditation it opens the solar plexus and brow chakras and helps to clear any blocked emotions.

CHEMICAL CONSTITUENTS OF ESSENTIAL OIL

TERPENES:

■ Monoterpenes: (alpha) pinene (3%), (beta) pinene (0.4–1%), myrcene (0.5–1.5%), (alpha) and (gamma) terpinene (7–8% and 14–18%), para-cymene (3–16%), limonene (1–3%), terpinolene

■ Sesquiterpenes: (beta) caryophyllene (1–2%), aromadendrene (2.75%), alloaromadendrene (9.4%), viridiflorene 1%, (alpha) and (delta) cadimenes (1.5–3%)

ALCOHOLS:

■ Monoterpenols (40–49%): terpinene 1-ol-4 (25–45%), (alpha) terpineol (3.5–5%), (alpha) terpineol, para cymenol (0.1%), cis and trans thujanol 4

■ Sesquiterpenols: globulol, viridiflorol

OXIDES:

■ Terpenic oxides: 1,4 cineole, 1,8 cineole (5–9%), epoxycaryophyllene ++

 ## BLENDS WELL WITH

Bergamot, Roman Chamomile, Lavender, Rosewood, Sandalwood, Pine, Rosemary, Cypress.

SAFETY PRECAUTIONS

No known ones.

ORIGANUM MAJORANA
Marjoram

Marjoram belongs to the family *Lamiaceae*, also known as *Labiatae*. It is grown in France, Spain, Morocco, Tunisia, Egypt, Germany, and Hungary.

ESSENTIAL OIL

The essential oil is obtained by steam distillation from the leaves. It is a Middle Note oil with a warming and loving temperament, a warm, spicy, floral, herbaceous scent, and a clear to pale amber color.

THE PLANT

Marjoram is a perennial herb which may reach 24–32 inches in height, with oblong, dark silver-green leaves, and a hairy stem which supports clusters of tiny pinkish-white flowers.

To the ancient Greeks, Sweet Marjoram was a funeral plant which would bring peace to the departed. Dedicated to Aphrodite, goddess of love and fertility, it was used as a symbol of eternal love to adorn the heads of young couples during marriage ceremonies. It was also cultivated by the ancient Egyptians for use in unguents, potions, medicines, and cookery. It was dedicated to the god Osiris, husband of Isis and king of the underworld. In the work of Dioscorides, a Greek physician and naturalist, Marjoram

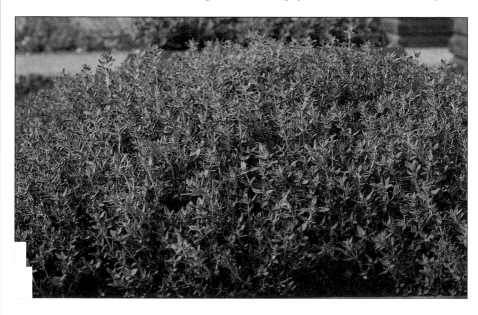

is referred to in the preparation of an ointment for warming and strengthening the nerves.

THERAPEUTIC EFFECTS

Positive charging molecules (2), analgesic, antiseptic, anti-spasmodic, calming, digestive, expectorant, hypotensor, laxative, parasympathetic nervous system tonic, sedative, vasodilator (improves circulation).

INDICATIONS AND COMMON USES

Therapeutic value ★★★

PHYSICAL SPHERE

■ **Respiratory system:** Marjoram is beneficial in synergistic formulations for bronchitis and colds.

■ **Digestive system:** in synergistic formulations for constipation and flatulence.

■ **Vascular system:** in synergistic formulations for hypertension.

■ **Joints and muscles:** good in synergistic formulations for arthritis, lower back pain due to muscle stiffness.

■ **Female reproductive system:** beneficial in synergistic formulations for menstrual pains.

PSYCHO-SPIRITUAL SPHERE

Essential oil of Marjoram is beneficial for those suffering from anxiety, insomnia, grief, and nervous tension.

CHEMICAL CONSTITUENTS OF ESSENTIAL OIL

TERPENES:
■ Monoterpenes (40%): (alpha) and (beta) pinenes, sabinene, myrcene, (alpha) and (gamma) terpinenes, paracimene, terpinolene, (alpha) and (beta) phellandrenes
■ Sesquiterpenes: caryophyllene, humulene

ALCOHOLS:
■ Monoterpenols (5%): linalol, terpineol 4, terpinene 1 ol 4, terpineol

PHENOLS:
■ Cis and trans thujanol-4

ESTERS:
■ Terpenic ester: terpenyl acetate, linalyl acetate, geranyl acetate

PHENOL METHYL ETHERS:
■ Trans anethole

BLENDS WELL WITH

Basil, Bergamot, Black Pepper, Roman Chamomile, Lemon, Orange, Pine, Spruce, Sea Pine, Tea Tree, Thyme Linalol, amongst others.

SAFETY PRECAUTIONS

None when used correctly.

PELARGONIUM GRAVEOLENS, PELARGONIUM X ASPERUM

Geranium

Geranium belongs to the family of the *Geraniaceae*. It is grown in Egypt, China, Reunion, and Russia.

ESSENTIAL OIL

The essential oil is obtained by steam distillation from the scented leaves. It is a Middle Note oil with a calming, warming and balancing temperament, a sweet, strong, rose-like, lively and floral scent, and a yellow to olive green color.

THE PLANT

These species of *Pelargonium* are perennial hairy shrubs, which grow to three feet in height. The leaves are pointed and serrated at the edges and very fragrant. The flowers are pink and small and also very fragrant.

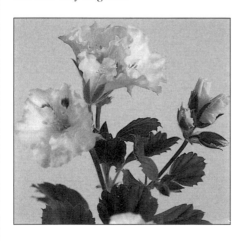

THERAPEUTIC EFFECTS

Positive charging molecules (2), anti-infectious: anti-bacterial and anti-fungal, analgesic, anti-inflammatory, anti-spasmodic, relaxant, astringent, cicatrisant, hemostratic ★★★, lymphatic system tonic, venous tonic.

INDICATIONS AND COMMON USES
Therapeutic value ★★★★

PHYSICAL SPHERE
■ **Skin:** beneficial in formulations for acne, eczema, fungal dermatitis, mature skin, oily skin, ringworm. For skincare preparations, Geranium is useful for inflamed, sluggish, congested, mature and oily skins.

■ **Endocrine glands:** it is a good adrenal stimulant.

■ **Urinary system:** good for fluid retention, urinary infections, swollen ankles.

■ **Vascular system:** helps in synergistic formulations for poor circulation, hemorrhoids (piles).

■ **Digestive system:** useful in formulations for the treatment of anal pruritus (itchiness), irritable bowel.

■ **Female reproductive system:** an eminently female oil beneficial in formulations for premenstrual tension and the menopause.

CHEMICAL CONSTITUENTS OF ESSENTIAL OIL

TERPENES:

■ Monoterpenes: (alpha) and (beta) phellandrenes (1–3.4%)

■ Sesquiterpenes: (alpha) copaene (0.35%), (delta) and (gamma) cadinenes (0.5%), guadiene, (alpha) and (beta) bourbonenes, guaiazulene

ALCOHOLS:

■ Aromatic: (beta) phenyl ethilic alcohol (0.8%)

■ Monoterpenic alcohols(60–68%): linalol (1.2%), (alpha) terpineol (0.25–2.2%), citronellol 33%, geraniol (25%), nerol (0.1%), menthol (1.2%)

ESTERS:

■ Terpenic esters (20–33%): citronelyl forniate (13%), gernayl forniate (1.8%), linalyl forniate, citronelyl acetate, geranyl acetate, citronellyl tiglate, geranyl tiglate, phenyl thyl tiglate (0.65%), citronellyl propionate (0.9%), geranyll propionate (0.6%), citronelyll butirate (0.9%), geranyl butirate

OXYDES:

■ 1,8—cineole (1.7%), cis and trans rose oxide, cis and trans linalol Oxydes

ALDEHYDES:

■ Neral, geranial (9.8%), citronellal (1.1%)

KETONES:

■ Alyphatic and terpenic: methylheptenone (0.5%), menthone and (–), isomenthone (7.5%), 1 nor bourbonanone, piperitone

SULPHURATED COMPOUNDS (S):

■ Di-methyl-sulfide

NITROGENATED OR AZOATED COMPOUNDS (N):

■ Citronellyl di-ethyl-amine

■ **Peripheral nerves:** neuralgia.

■ **Joints:** has been shown to be of benefit in formulations for osteoarthritis.

PSYCHO-SPIRITUAL SPHERE

Geranium provides help and calm; it is refreshing to the psyche, and feeds and balances psycho-spiritual needs. Geranium has the ability to improve anxiety and depression, and give emotional protection. It is very uplifting and a tonic to the nervous system. A balancing oil, not too sedative or too stimulating—a good balancing oil for tiredness, general fatigue, and convalescence. In meditation it opens the solar plexus and heart chakras.

BLENDS WELL WITH

Bergamot, Cypress, Neroli, Rose, Rosewood, Sandalwood, Lavender.

SAFETY PRECAUTIONS

Geranium is a very safe oil when the correct dosages are utilized.

PINUS SYLVESTRIS

Scots Pine

Scots Pine belongs to the family *Coniferae*, also known as *Abietaceae*. It grows in Austria, Italy, the eastern United States, Russia, and Yugoslavia.

ESSENTIAL OIL

The essential oil is obtained by steam distillation of the needles and small branches. It is a Middle Note oil with a warming and soothing temperament, an aromatic, balsamic, fresh turpentine-like scent, and is colorless to pale yellow.

THE PLANT

Scots Pine is an evergreen tree

CHEMICAL CONSTITUENTS OF ESSENTIAL OIL

TERPENES:
■ Monoterpenes (high percentage): (alpha) and (beta) pinenes (40 and 12.9%), 9-10-limonene (20–30%)
■ Sesquiterpenes: longifolene, (beta) caryophyllene

ALCOHOLS:
■ Monoterpenols: borneol (12%)
■ Sesquiterpenols: (alpha) cadimol

ESTERS:
■ 1–15%: Terpenic esters: bornyl acetate

which grows up to 99 feet in height, with a reddish-brown bark and pale brown cones, the source of pine kernels.

THERAPEUTIC EFFECTS

Positive charging molecules (2), antiseptic, anti-fungal, decongestant: lymphatic, uterine and ovarian. Hormone-like due to its stimulating effect on the adeno-hypophysis, anti-diabetic effect: through the pituitary-pancreatic hormonal reflex axis, cortision like ★★★★ effect through the pituitary-cortico-adrenal hormonal reflex axis, sexual stimulant effect through the pituitary-ovrian or pituitary-testicular hormonal reflex axis, neurotonic and hypertensive.

INDICATIONS AND COMMON USES
Therapeutic value ★★★★

PHYSICAL SPHERE
■ **Joints and muscles:** Scots Pine is beneficial in formulations for arthritis.
■ **Respiratory system:** Scots Pine is beneficial in formulations for asthma, bronchitis. sinusitis.
■ **Nervous system:** in formulations for multiple sclerosis.
■ **Female reproductive system:** Scots Pine is beneficial in some formulations

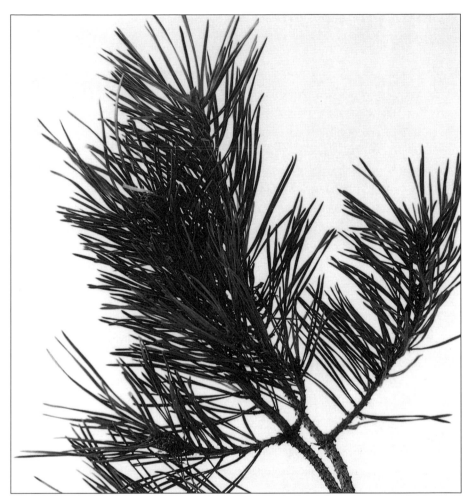

for the treatment of uterine congestion.

PSYCHO-SPIRITUAL SPHERE

Scots Pine is beneficial in formulations for asthenia (lack of physical and mental energy).

BLENDS WELL WITH

True Lavender, Lavandin, Patchouli, Black Pepper, Spruce, Lemon, Petitgrain, Rosemary.

SAFETY PRECAUTIONS

No known side effects if used correctly.

ROSA DAMASCENA

Bulgarian Rose

Bulgarian Rose belongs to the family *Rosaceae*. It is one of the most beautifully scented essential oils and one of the most expensive as it takes 60,000 Roses to obtain an ounce of Rose oil. There are three varieties of Roses used for the extraction of the oil *Rosa damascena*. They grow mainly in Bulgaria, Tunisia, France, and Turkey.

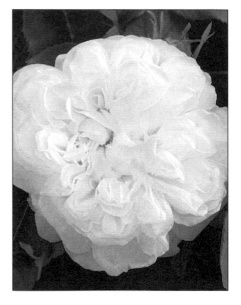

 ## ESSENTIAL OIL

The oil is obtained by steam distillation of the petals of *Rosa damascena*. It is a Middle to Top Note oil with a moist, grounding, warm and mothering temperament, with a delicate, gentle, sweet floral scent, and a dark to pale yellow color.

 ## THE PLANT

The Rose bush grows up to four feet. The flowers are deep magenta pink but it may occasionally have white flowers.

The Rose was called the "queen of flowers" by the Greek bard Sappho, and in Greek mythology the Rose was believed to have originated from the blood of Adonis. The history of aromatics is deeply linked with the Rose, as it is said that Cleopatra sailed down the Nile with the sails of her ship soaked in Rose oil, so that the beautiful aroma would precede her and announce her arrival. It is also thought that she used Rose oil abundantly in her beauty routine.

Rose oil was the first oil to be distilled by the Arab physician Avicenna in the eleventh century and is still one of the best-loved essential oils and flowers.

 ## THERAPEUTIC EFFECTS

Negative charging molecules (2), aphrodisiac, anti-depressant, anti-inflammatory, antiseptic, anti-spasmodic, astringent, emenagogue, hemostatic, hepatic (good for the liver), sedative, laxative, depurative (helps inner digestive) cleansing, uterine tonic.

CHEMICAL CONSTITUENTS OF ESSENTIAL OIL

TERPENES:

- Monoterpenes 1%: (alpha) pinene 1%, (beta) pinene 1%, myrcene 1%, limonene 1%, sabinene 1%
- Sesquiterpenes 2%: caryophylene 1%, guaiene 1%, humulene 1%, D germacrene 1%, bulnesene 1%, cadimene 1%, bourbonene 1%, elemene 1%

ALCOHOLS:

- Monoterpenic alcohols: 62% are formed by the following three: citronellol also known as rhodinol 28–35%; geeaniol 15–20%; nerol 7–10%
- The other monoterpenic alcohols found in Rose are: linalol, terpineol 4.1%, terpineol 1%
- Sesquiterpenic alcohols: farnesol 1%

PHENOLS:

- Eugenol 1%

ALDEHYDES 1%:

- Geranial

ESTERS:

- Geranyl acetate 1–3%, citronellyl acetate 1%, phenyl-ethyl acetate 1%, citronellyl forniate 1%, phenyl-ethyl isovalerate 1%, neryl acetate 1%, geranyl acetate 1%

OXYDES:

- Cis and trans rose oxyde

KETONES:

- Traces of: damascenone (C13), damasone (C13)

ETHERS 3%:

- Methyl eugenol 3%

ACIDS 1%:

- Benzoin acid, valeric acid, acetic acid

INDICATIONS AND COMMON USES

Therapeutic value ★★★★

PHYSICAL SPHERE

- **Skin:** Rose is beneficial in formulations for ageing skin, mature skin and sensitive skin.
- **Digestive system:** beneficial in formulations for nausea and constipation.
- **Reproductive system:** good in formulations for treating frigidity, impotence, irregular periods, leucorrhea, infertility of unexplained origin, and uterine disorders.

PSYCHO-SPIRITUAL SPHERE

Rose is beneficial for those suffering from insomnia, nervous tension, tension headaches and extreme bereavement and grief.

 ## BLENDS WELL WITH

Sandalwood, Neroli, Jasmine, Rosewood, Geranium, Bergamot, and all citruses.

SAFETY PRECAUTIONS

Rose is a very safe oil when used correctly.

ROSMARINUS OFFICINALIS CAMPHORIFERUM

Rosemary

Rosemary belongs to the family *Lamiaceae*, also known as *Labiatae*. It is grown for oil production in Corsica, France, Morocco, Spain, and Tunisia.

ESSENTIAL OIL

The essential oil is obtained by steam distillation from the leaves and twigs. It is a Top Note oil with a warm, stimulating, uplifting temperament, a refreshing, herby scent with woody undertones, and is a clear colorless liquid.

THE PLANT

Rosemary is an evergreen shrub, growing up to six feet in height, with needle shaped, silver leaves and blue flowers. This herb was very highly regarded by all the ancient civilizations. Traces were found in the first dynasty Egyptian tombs; the Hebrews used it as part of the bitter herbs on the Passover table and in other rituals involving foods; the Maya and Inca civilizations used it as part of their religious ceremonies; the Greek physician Hippocrates recommended Rosemary for liver and spleen disorders; and during the sixteenth century it was used by the Swiss physician and alchemist Paracelsus.

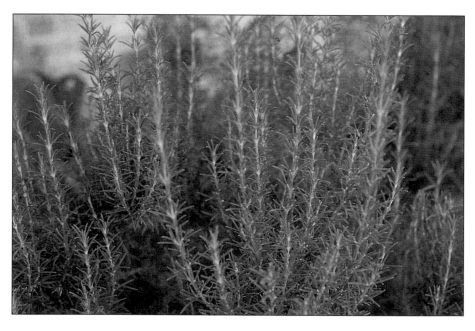

During the thirteenth century, a Spanish physician and alchemist, Dr. Arnaldo de Villanueva, managed to distill oil of Rosemary. In his writings he praised the value of his oils and waters of Rosemary, quoting their stimulating effect on the brain. The story of the "ugly" Hungarian queen who drank Rosemary water and became beautiful and married a handsome Polish king is part of the folklore associated with this herb. In 1370 a refreshing Eau de Cologne, known as Hungarian Water, was first marketed in honor of Queen Elizabeth of Hungary, containing oil of Rosemary in its formulation.

CHEMICAL CONSTITUENTS OF ESSENTIAL OIL

TERPENES:
- Monoterpenes: (alpha) pinene, (beta) pinene, camphene
- Sesquiterpenes: (delta) caryophyllene

ALCOHOLS:
- Monoterpenols: borneol

ESTERS:
- Terpenic esters: nonyl acetate

OXYDES:
- Terpenic: cineole

KETONES:
- Monoterpenones: camphone

THERAPEUTIC EFFECTS

Positive charging molecules (2), anti-catarrhal, expectorant, mucolytic, bactericide, fungicide. Good for the liver, aids concentration and memory.

INDICATIONS AND COMMON USES

Therapeutic value ★★★

PHYSICAL SPHERE

- **Respiratory system:** Rosemary is beneficial in formulations for bronchitis, otitis, sinusitis.
- **Genito-urinary system:** beneficial in formulations for cystitis.
- **Digestive system:** good in formulations for fermentative enterocolitis.
- **Nervous system:** Rosemary is beneficial in formulations for multiple sclerosis (used as a secondary oil).

PSYCHO-SPIRITUAL SPHERE

Rosemary is beneficial for those suffering from depression, anxiety, anguish, and emotional numbness. In meditation, it opens the heart chakra, clears confusion, eliminates doubt, and lifts exhaustion.

BLENDS WELL WITH

Geranium, Lavender, Lemon, Sandalwood, Juniper, Tea Tree, Ravensara, Thyme Linalol.

SAFETY PRECAUTIONS

None at recommended dosages.

ROSMARINUS OFFICINALIS VERBENONIFERUM

Rosemary verbenone

This belongs to the family *Lamiaceae*, also known as *Labiatae*. The essential oil of Rosemary is produced nowadays in France and Spain.

Rosemary is a Top Note oil with a warm, stimulating temperament, a refreshing, herby scent with apple undertones. It is a clear colorless liquid.

ESSENTIAL OIL

This essential oil is obtained by steam distillation of the leaves and twigs.

THE PLANT

Rosemary is an evergreen shrub, growing up to six feet in height,

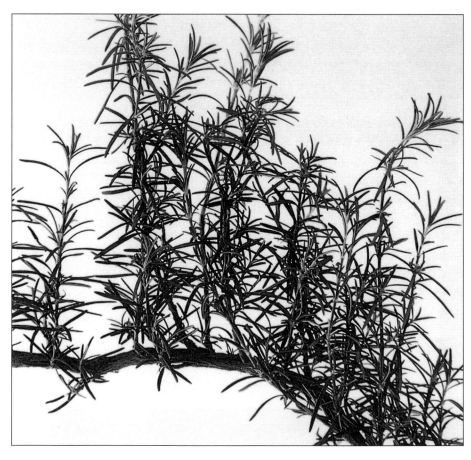

CHEMICAL CONSTITUENTS OF ESSENTIAL OIL

TERPENES:
- Monoterpenes: pinene (alpha), pinene (beta), camphene, myrcenc, limonenc, terpinene (alpha), terpinolene

SESQUITERPENES:
- caryopphylene (beta)

ALCOHOLS:
- Monoterpenols: Borneol

ESTERS:
- Terpenic: bornyl acetate

KETONES
- Monoterpenones: Verbenone 15-37%, camphone

OXYDES:
- Terpenic: 1-6 cineole

with needle-shaped silver leaves and blue flowers.

Regarded very highly by all ancient civilizations, traces were found in first-dynasty Egyptian tombs. Hebrews used it as part of the bitter herbs on the Passover table and other rituals, involving foods. The Maya and Inca civilizations used it as part of their religious ceremonies. The Greek physician Hippocrates recommended it for liver and spleen disorders, during the sixteenth century by the Swiss physician and alchemist Teophrastus Bombastus von Hohenheim, better known as Paracelsus.

THERAPEUTIC EFFECTS

Hepatic, digestive, carminative, cicatrisant, lipophilic.

INDICATIONS AND COMMON USES
Therapeutic value ★★★

PHYSICAL SPHERE
- **Digestive system:** liver problems due to over-eating, gallbladder disfunctions.
- **Skin:** good for acne, psoriasis and skin allergies.

PSYCHO-SPIRITUAL SPHERE
This is a very special oil: it is good for meditation to open the third chakra, it works balancing the solar plexus and helps to alleviate depression and tensions.

BLENDS WELL WITH

Bergamot, Lavender, Lemon, Geranium.

SAFETY PRECAUTIONS

Due to its high ketone content it should only be used when specifically recommended.

SANTALUM ALBUM
Sandalwood

Sandalwood belongs to the *Santalaceae* family. The essential oil of Sandalwood is produced in the East Indies and the Indian archipelago, where the plant grows wildly in the areas of Mysore and Madras. However, other species, either cultivated or wild, have been identified in Java, Borneo, New Caledonia, and Australia.

ESSENTIAL OIL
The oil is produced by a process of steam distillation from the heartwood. Sandalwood is a Middle to Base Note oil, with a calming, comforting temperament and a characteristic woody, balsamic odor. The scent is faint but lovely, persistent and long lasting. The oil is a pale yellow to nearly clear in color.

THE PLANT
White or citrine Sandalwood is a small shrub reaching 24–60 feet in height. It is considered a parasitic tree because after germination its roots bury themselves in those of neighboring trees from which they extract minerals and water. This eventually causes the surrounding vegetation to perish. As the tree grows, the oil develops in the roots and the heartwood. The latter only starts developing after 15 years of growth. The tree is found in open, dry places of the southern highlands of southern India and the Malaysian Archipelago.

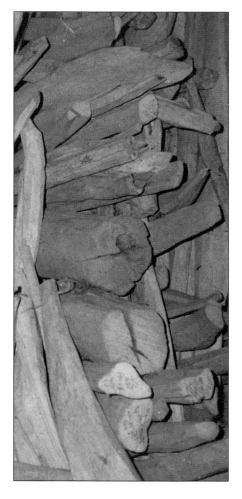

The Sandalwood tree only becomes fully mature after 60 years. The amount of oil produced in trees of less than 30 years of age is very small, and therefore these young trees are never harvested unless they are affected by disease.

THERAPEUTIC EFFECTS

Negative charging molecules (1), anti-depressant, antiseptic (genito-urinary), astringent (tightens the pores), cardiotonic (heart tonic), decongestant, diuretic, expectorant, lymphatic decongestant, sedative, venous decongestant.

INDICATIONS AND COMMON USES
Therapeutic value ★★★★

PHYSICAL SPHERE
■ **Skin:** Sandalwood has traditionally been used in blends for acne and mature, ageing skin.
■ **Respiratory system:** helps with bronchitis, especially chronic bronchitis, catarrhs, and coughs.
■ **Nervous system:** sciatica.
■ **Genito-urinary system:** a beneficial oil for chronic cystitis, piuria (pus in the urine), prostatitis.
■ **Female reproductive system:** Sandalwood oil is a useful part of blends of essential oils for methritis and other menstrual problems.
■ **Circulation:** helps in the treatment of hemorrhoids, varicose veins.

PSYCHO-SPIRITUAL SPHERE
Sandalwood is beneficial as part of synergistic formulations for treating

CHEMICAL CONSTITUENTS OF ESSENTIAL OIL

TERPENES:
■ Sesquiterpenes (5%): (alpha) and (beta) santalenes, epi- (beta) santalene, (alpha) curcumene, (beta) farnesene

ALCOHOLS:
■ Sesquiterpenols (90–93%): (alpha) and (beta) santalol (67–90%)*, epi (beta) santalol (4.5%), trans (beta) santalol, lanceol, trans (alpha) bergamotol, tere-santalol (minor component), tri-cyclic-sesquiterpenic alcohols

ALDEHYDES:
■ Sesquiterpenals: tere-santalal, nor-tri-cyclo-santalal

ACIDS:
■ Carboxylic acids: nor-tricilo-santalic acid, tere-santalic acid

depression, especially when it is coupled with nervous conditions such as anxiety, stress, and tension.

BLENDS WELL WITH

Bergamot, Lavender, Lemon, Rosewood, Ginger, Orange, Neroli, Patchouli, Pine, Rose.

SAFETY PRECAUTIONS

At therapeutic dosages this oil has no known contraindications.

ZINGIBER OFFICINALIS
Ginger

Ginger belongs to the *Zingiberaceae* family. It is grown in India, the West Indies, and Sri Lanka.

THE ESSENTIAL OIL

The essential oil is obtained by steam distillation from the rhizomes of the rootlets. It is a Base Note oil with a warming and balancing temperament, and has a spicy, lively scent, which is equally loved by both sexes. It is pale yellow in color.

THE PLANT

Ginger is a perennial plant, a native of those countries which have a tropical climate, and can reach up to 20–39 feet in height, with lanceolate leaves and tuberous thick rhizomes, which give rise to reed-like stems and yellow flowers with purple patterns.

Ginger has been used for centuries in China, India, the Far East, and South America for both culinary and medicinal purposes.

THERAPEUTIC EFFECTS

Positive charging molecules (2), antiseptic, stomachic, digestive tonic, aphrodisiac, analgesic, expectorant, warming, anti-rheumatic, sudorific (increases sweating).

INDICATIONS AND COMMON USES
Therapeutic value ★★★

PHYSICAL SPHERE

■ **Joints and muscles:** essential oil of Ginger is beneficial in formulations for arthritis, aching muscles, rheumatism.

■ **Respiratory system:** a beneficial oil in formulations for coughs and colds, chronic bronchitis.

■ **Digestive system:** in loss of appetite, flatulence, heartburn, constipation, diarrhea. Gently massage the abdominal area with a three percent blend of essential oil of Ginger in Sweet Almond oil.

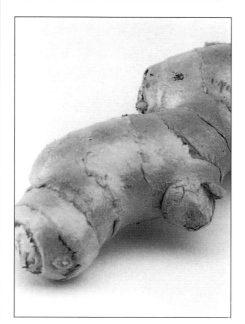

CHEMICAL CONSTITUENTS OF ESSENTIAL OIL

TERPENES:

■ Monoterpenes: (alpha) pinene, camphene, (beta) pinene, myrcene, limonene, (beta) phelandrene

■ Sesquiterpenes: cyclosativene, cyclo-copa camphene, copaene, sesquithujene, (beta) ylangene, (beta) elemene, trans (beta) farnesene, (beta) caryophylene, selina 4,11 diene, selina 3,11 diene, (alpha) anphorphene, 10 epizonarene, cis (gamma) bisabolene, zingiberene, (beta) sesquiphelandrene, gernacrene B, D calamenene

HYDROCARBONS:

■ Aliphatic and aromatic: Undecaene, Dodecaene, Hexadecaene, Toloene, Para cimene

ALCOHOLS:

■ Aliphatic alcohols: 2 methyl–butanol, 2 heptanol, 2 nonanol

■ Monoterpenic alcohols: linalol (0.6%), citronellol (2%)

AROMATIC MOLECULES:

■ Cuminic alcohol

■ Sesquiterpenic alcohols: nerolidol, elemol, cis sesqui-bissabolene hydrate, (beta) bisabolol, zingiberenol, (beta) eudesmol, trans (beta) sesquiphellandrol

ALDEHYDES:

■ Alyphatic aldehydes: butanal, 2 methyl butanal, 3 methyl butanal, pentanal, pentalal

■ Monoterpenic aldehydes: citronellal, myrtenal, phellandral, neral, geranial

KETONES:

■ Aliphatic ketones: acetone, 2 hexanone, 2 heptanone, 2 nonanone, methyl heptanone

■ Monoterpenic ketones: cryptone, carvotanacetone

PSYCHO-SPIRITUAL SPHERE

Ginger is a good oil for those lacking in motivation and initiative, and for those who lack the confidence to achieve their potential. It is also a beneficial boost, aiding will power and energy levels, and can help those suffering with physical and psychological impotence. Ginger provides grounding and has a warming effect where cold and air prevail. In meditation it opens the solar plexus and brow chakras.

BLENDS WELL WITH

Eucalyptus Radiata, Lemon, Orange, Sandalwood, Frankincense, Patchouli.

SAFETY PRECAUTIONS

Do not use neat undiluted essential oil of Ginger on the skin as it may cause sensitivity.

OTHER ESSENTIAL OILS

Aniba rosaeodora var *amazonica*
ROSEWOOD
Rosewood belongs to the *Lauraceae* family. It grows in Brazil and the Amazon rainforest.

■ **The essential oil** is extracted by stem distillation of the wood. It is a Middle Note oil with a warm, caring temperament, a sweet, spicy, floral, and lightly woody scent, and a pale yellow to brownish color.

■ **Therapeutic effects:** Rosewood is anti-infectious, anti-bacterial, anti-fungal, anti-parasitic, anti-viral, stimulant tonic.

■ **Therapeutic value** ★★★

■ **Physical sphere:** Rosewood is beneficial for the respiratory and the female reproductive systems.

■ **Psycho-spiritual sphere:** beneficial for asthenia and depression.

Safety: safe when used correctly.

Eucalyptus radiata
EUCALYPTUS RADIATA
This belongs to the Myrtaceae family. The essential oil is produced in Australia.

■ **The essential oil** is obtained by steam distillation from the Eucalyptus leaves. It is a Top Note oil with a warming, clearing temperament, a camphor-like and slightly woody scent, and a clear color.

■ **Therapeutic effects:** Eucalyptus Radiata is antiseptic, antiviral, anti-asthenic, anti-catarrhal, anti-inflammatory, and an expectorant.

■ **Therapeutic value** ★★★

■ **Physical sphere:** it is good for treating some types of acne, the respiratory, female reproductive, and immune systems.

■ **Psycho-spiritual sphere:** it clears and opens the heart and throat chakras.

Safety: a safe oil when utilized correctly.

Lavandula intermedia/hybrida
LAVANDIN
Lavandin is a hybrid of *Lavandula angustifolia* and *Lavandula latifolia*.

■ **The essential oil** is produced by steam distillation of the flowering tops. It is a Top Note oil with a warming, balancing temperament, a gentle, lively floral scent, and a clear to pale yellow color.

■ **Therapeutic effects:** it is anti-infectious, anti-bacterial, anti-fungal, anti-catarrhal, an expectorant, general tonic.

■ **Therapeutic value** ★★★

■ **Physical sphere:** beneficial for the digestive and respiratory systems.

■ **Psycho-spiritual sphere:** it is a very good oil for general asthenia.

Safety: a very safe oil if used correctly at the right dosages.

Trachyspermum anni
AJOWAN
Ajowan belongs to the *Umbelliferae* family, also known as the *Apiacae* family. It originates from Egypt, and is cultivated in Southwest Asia and the Mediterranean.

■ **The essential oil** is obtained by steam distillation from the dried and crushed

SPECIAL NOTES

1 Throughout this chapter on essential oils, their uses and properties, a star system has been used to indicate their therapeutic value.

2 The phrase "negative charging molecules" refers to the potential that the essential oil molecules have, when in contact with cells, to release electrons and bind any excessive and potentially damaging ions (free radicals).

3 The phrase "positive charging molecules" refers to the potential that essential oil molecules have, when in contact with cells, to bind any excessive and potentially damaging negative ions.

4 Both of the above phrases, "positive charging" and "negative charging molecules," refer to the electrical polarity and the effect that the molecules will have when entering the cells and the body.

fruits. Ajowan is a Top to Middle Note oil with a warming, balancing temperament, a spicy, fruity scent, and a color ranging from colorless to brownish yellow.

■ The plant is a herbaceous winter annual, growing up to three feet in height with white flowers. The fruit is ovoid and small.

■ **Therapeutic effects:** Ajowan is analgesic, antiseptic, antispasmodic, carminative, a digestive stimulant.

■ **Therapeutic value**: ★★

■ **Physical sphere:** Ajowan is beneficial for the digestive and skeletal systems, and the peripheral nerves.

■ **Psycho-spiritual sphere:** Ajowan is used for treating hysteria and depression. It opens the root chakra and solar plexus chakra, and helps remove fear.

■ **Safety:** may irritate skin; use only at low dilutions of 1.5 percent. Do not use in pregnancy and in children under 12 years.

PURCHASING AND STORING ESSENTIAL OILS

■ Always purchase essential oils from a well-known supplier who can offer certificates of purity and quality if required.

■ The Latin name and place of origin of the oils should be printed on the supplier's list. However, there are always variations between crops, and a quality oil may not have the same scent year after year.

■ A good oil should be as natural as possible and grown wild in its own habitat.

■ Essential oils should always be supplied in dark glass bottles with insert droppers, and clearly labeled with the English and Botanical names, the amount contained in the bottle, the batch number, and date.

■ You should store essential oils in a cool, dark cabinet or room.

■ Never prepare formulations near an open flame; essential oils are volatile and thus flammable.

■ Do not use essential oils in a stuffy room; you may inhale too much.

■ Avoid any contact with your eyes.

■ Some oils have an irritant effect on the skin when applied neat. This is transient in a majority of cases and no damage has been reported from accidentally spilling one or two drops of an undiluted oil on the skin.

THE BASE CARRIER OILS

In order to be able to use essential oils correctly and get the maximum benefit from their use, they have to be made into formations which utilize a carrier or base, usually a vegetable oil. However, it may also be a vegetable gel or cream.

FATTY OILS

All fatty oils have a number of characteristics that make them alike: they contain fatty acids and are insoluble in water, being lighter than water. Generally they solidify at temperatures below 32°F, while they remain as liquids at temperatures above 32°F.

In old medical manuscripts which document early expeditions by explorers to the Indies, we can read about the contents of the first aid kits of the physicians or barbers who accompanied the expeditions. Every kit contained oils, animal fat, pink honey and bezoar stones (regurgitated by llamas, vicunas, and deer, all of them ruminant animals), which had anti-poisonous properties and were held in great esteem. In those ancient times, fatty oils were greatly utilized by healers and sharmans.

TYPES OF CARRIER OILS

The main carrier oils are vegetable fatty oils, which are cold expressed from nuts and seeds. For example, we have Sweet Almond oil, Apricot kernel oil, Peach kernel oil, Wheatgerm oil, Avocado oil, and Rosehip oil amongst others.

Fatty oils are obtained from seeds by the following process: first the seeds are cleaned thoroughly with machines to which brushes are attached. The seeds are then placed in grinding and pounding mills. The pulp is wrapped in linens and placed in large pressing machines. The expression is carried out cold or at very low temperatures, which gives a very good quality oil although the yield is lower than fatty oils that are obtained from hot expression.

USES OF FATTY OILS

Fatty oils have also been used on their own merits in massage since ancient times. They have many nourishing and healing properties for wound healing and in skin care. There are also some liquid waxes, such as the one extracted from the Jojoba nut, which can be used as carriers, not forgetting gels such as the one extracted from the Aloe Vera cactus, which can also be successfully utilized as a vehicle for essential oils.

SWEET ALMOND OIL

Sweet Almond oil is extracted by cold expression from *Prunus amygdalus*. In the process of extraction, first the seeds are separated from their hard husks and then they are cold pressed. Sweet Almond oil has the characteristic of being rich in unsaturated fatty acids and vitamins A, B1, B6 and E. Thus it has a healing effect on the skin and is very good for using on various skin types. It is absorbed very quickly by the skin and does not leave a fatty residue when massaged.

APRICOT KERNEL OIL

Apricot kernel oil is another very useful carrier which has a light, pale yellow color and no smell. It is used in many blends for the body and face and has the quality of penetrating into the skin very quickly due to its low viscosity.

WHEATGERM OIL

The botanical name of Wheatgerm is *Triticum estivum*. This oil is very rich in vitamin E and thus has an orange color. It is a very viscous oil and has an antioxidant effect. It protects the skin and the cardiovascular system from the harm caused by free radicals which it counteracts. For aromatherapy massage treatments, Wheatgerm oil should be added to one of the other vegetable base oils in a proportion of five to ten percent.

AVOCADO OIL

The botanical name of the Avocado is *Persea gratisima*. This oil is obtained by cold expression of the seed of the Avocado. It is very rich in vitamin A, and in lower quantities also contains vitamins B, C, D, E, H, and K. Due to this it is very effective as an anti-ageing carrier oil. Avocado oil is very viscous and should also be used as part of an aromatherapy essential oil formulation in proportions of up to

15 percent with either Sweet Almond or Apricot kernel oils.

ROSEHIP OIL

This oil is known as *Rosa rubiginosa* or *Rosa mosqueta Chile*. It is a very good base oil, obtained from the seeds of the Rosehip, and has the unique quality of containing the same polyunsaturated fatty acids as the human skin, namely arachidonic acid, linoleic acid, and alpha linolenic acid, of which the last two are particularly beneficial for their regenerating properties of the human skin. Rosehip oil is very useful for treating scars and stretch marks, and also for the treatment of scarring following various surgeries when it aids a speedy recovery. It may be used in a 50:50 dilution with any of the other carrier oils or, if treating extensive scarring, it can be used undiluted with the appropriate choice of essential oils.

JOJOBA OIL

From the plant known as *Simondsia sinensis*, Jojoba oil is a liquid wax, rather than a fatty oil. It is golden yellow in color and has a light smell. It is obtained by cold expression of the small, round, brown nuts. Jojoba oil contains many vitamins and trace elements and is an excellent carrier that leaves the skin silky and soft and is absorbed very quickly through its layers. A very good base oil for aromatherapy massage is made up with 50 percent Jojoba oil added to 50 percent Rosehip oil, as this has a very effective and therapeutic anti-ageing effect.

CHAPTER THREE

AROMATHERAPY TREATMENTS

An aromatherapy treatment may consist of various modalities or types of treatment. For example, a long-term treatment may involve more than one specific treatment at any given time. It may consist of either an aromatherapy massage treatment, which utilizes the carefully prepared blend of essential oils and base oils chosen for the person's individual needs following a consultation with a qualified professional aromatherapist, or a home treatment utilizing the techniques described below and a blend of oils prepared by careful choice and with professional advice whenever required. In addition to the aromatherapy massage treatment, there are a number of other methods of treatment which are also very effective and beneficial if adequately chosen. Amongst these are the following ones.

Below: an aromatherapy massage may be relaxing and soothing, or energizing and revitalizing for the recipient.

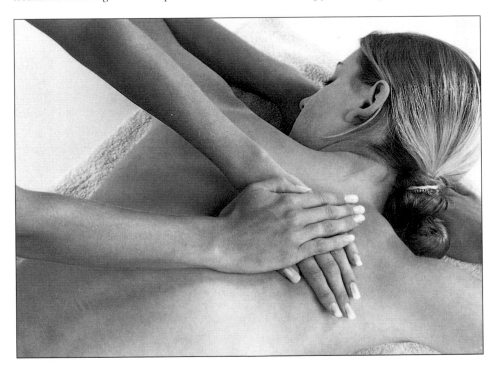

BATHS

An aromatherapy bath is a very effective method of self-treatment, which may be taken either in the morning on rising, in the evening before retiring, or at any other time when it is deemed necessary. An aromatic bath is prepared as follows:

1 Ensure that you have a quiet, undisturbed half an hour or an hour by making sure that your children are being looked after, the phones are on hold, and any other foreseen interruptions are taken care of.

2 Choose one to three of your favorite and appropriate essential oils.

3 Make a blend with two drops of each essential oil in a teaspoon of carrier oil— either Sweet Almond oil or Apricot kernel oil is a good choice.

4 Run your bath at the temperature you feel comfortable with; the bath should be pleasantly warm, not hot, as a hot bath may be very uncomfortable.

5 When your tub is full to the appropriate level and you are ready to get in, pour the blend of essential oils into the water and swish it around. The main reason for adding the blend only at this point and not when turning on the tap as you would do with other bath preparations is that, due to the volatility or capability for evaporating in contact with air, if adding the blend at the beginning you would end up with your essential oils all over your bathroom and not in your bath.

6 Do not use detergents or soaps when having an aromatic bath; this is not a cleansing but a therapeutic bath. Depending on your choice of oils, it may be relaxing, revitalizing, or stimulating; it may be used to help insomnia and depression as well as for many other purposes.

7 Try to remain in the water for about 20 minutes, which is the optimum time for your bodily systems to absorb and gain the most benefit from the essential oils.

8 When the time has elapsed, gently get out of your bath, dry yourself, relax for a few minutes, and then get dressed. Continue your planned activities, either to go out or to get ready for a night's sleep.

AROMATHERAPY COMPRESSES

An aromatherapy compress is a very useful treatment tool for many aches and pains. A compress may be either hot or cold

Below: an aromatherapy compress can treat aches and pains.

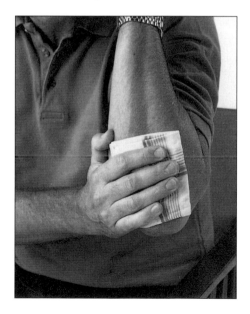

PREPARING A COMPRESS

This is a very simple procedure and it only requires the following materials:

- A clean piece of lint or a handkerchief
- A bowl of either cold or boiling water
- The chosen essential oils

depending on the need, e.g. when you have sprained your ankle or your child has bumped his head, a cold aromatic compress is an ideal treatment to help to alleviate the pain and reduce the swelling which has developed. However, when suffering from period pains or abdominal cramps due to indigestion, a hot aromatic compress is a blessing. To choose the oils required in each circumstance, refer to the description of each essential oil in Chapter Two.

1 Soak the cloth in the water and wring it out thoroughly.

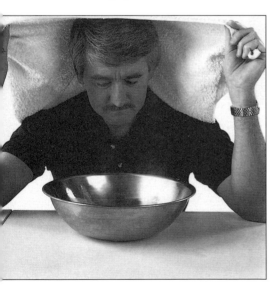

2 Add eight drops of your chosen oil to the bowl of water; you will observe that the oil will float on the surface.

3 Fold the cloth in the shape required to fit on the affected area and gently place the cloth on the surface of the water to collect the essential oil droplets.

4 Immediately place the cloth on the area requiring treatment.

5 To ensure that the compress remains in contact with the affected area, cover and wrap plastic wrap around the area.

6 Replace the compress after eight or twelve hours.

7 Depending on the severity of the damage you may need to continue this treatment for two or three days.

Note: the oils specially recommended for bruising, sport injuries, and sprains are Lavender for mild injuries, and Immortelle for the more severe ones. In the case of period cramps, a hot compress with essential oil of Geranium is very effective.

AROMATHERAPY INHALATIONS

Aromatic inhalations are a very effective method of aromatherapy treatment for respiratory ailments, coughs, colds, sinus problems, headaches due to sinus problems, and other minor ailments.

1 Place some drops of your chosen blend of essential oils, usually three to four, on the boiling water.

Left: when inhaling, use a towel to cover your head and lean over the steam, breathing in deeply.

2 Cover your head with the towel and lean over the steam, breathing deeply and regularly through the nose to obtain the maximum benefit.

3 If you have a facial sauna, place only three to four drops of essential oil on the water that is contained in the steamer compartment, then place your face in the opening and breathe deeply.

Note: should you have a very congested and stuffy nose, keep trying to breathe through your nose until the hot steam and the therapeutic effect of the essential oil alleviate the congestion. Continue with this treatment for between 10 and 15 minutes and repeat three to four times a day depending on your need.

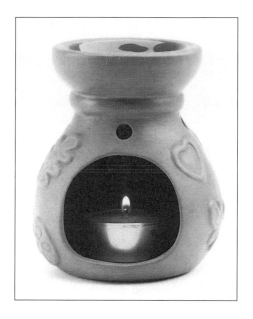

Above: ceramic diffusers diffuse an essential oil in a room.

AROMATHERAPY DIFFUSERS AND VAPORIZERS

In order to diffuse an essential oil in a room, either to create a special atmosphere or to prevent the spread of air droplets which disseminate and help to spread colds and other viral infections, specially designed aromatherapy vaporizers may be used. These are of various types, and the most commonly used ones are as follows:

■ **Ceramic diffusers** contain a night light as a source of heat and a well or a saucer, which is above the source of heat and is filled with water on which a few drops of the required blend of essential oils are placed. These can last for about eight or ten hours, depending on the depth of the well and the proximity to the night light.

■ **Vaporizers** are specially designed glass essential oil containers attached to an electric pump which blows cold air and diffuses the essential oil molecules into the atmosphere of the room. Some of these also have special glass attachments which direct the stream of essential oil molecules very close to the nose. Vaporizers must be used in conjunction with a qualified therapist and specific individually tailored formulations and blends.

■ **Aroma stone and electric diffusers** also heat the essential oil and diffuse it into the room. They are specially designed and are plugged in to the mains. They are marginally safer than the night light diffusers as there is no open flame; sometimes these diffusers are used in hospices and hospital wards.

AROMATHERAPY MASSAGE TREATMENT

Massage is one of the oldest treatments utilized to "make people feel better." It encourages the body to heal itself, and restores balance to all cells, tissues, and organs. The healing powers of touch and massage have been recognized since antiquity by all ancient civilizations, including the Chinese, Egyptians, Incas, Maya, Indians, Hebrews, Greeks, and Romans. Traditional healers worldwide have been aware of the beneficial effects of touch. It is known that some 25,000 years ago Hippocrates, the father of medicine, whose Hippocratic Oath is still taken today by conventional doctors on their graduation day, is quoted as insisting that "a physician must be experienced in many things but assured in rubbing, which can bind a joint that is too loose and loosen a joint that is too rigid."

Massage treatments suffered a severe setback in the Middle Ages when the Christian Church banned this kind of treatment relating it to "pleasures of the flesh." However, in 1813, a Swedish gymnast, Per Henrik Ling, devised a massage system which combined passive gymnastic movements with some Chinese massage techniques. The Royal Central Institute of Stockholm lent its name to this system, which has since been known as Swedish massage and has been the basis of many present day Western massage practices.

HOW DOES AN AROMATHERAPY MASSAGE WORK?

How is it that we are able to influence the functioning of our internal organs by stroking and kneading our skin? Generally, it is very seldom that all parts of our body work in such a wonderful synchronicity

EFFECTS OF AROMATHERAPY MASSAGE

Regular aromatherapy massage treatments are exceptionally beneficial to those who lead sedentary and/or stressful lives. The effects of an aromatherapy massage on the body systems are many:

■ It increases the nourishment and oxygen supply to the tissues by increasing and regulating blood circulation.

■ It enhances lymph drainage.

■ It stimulates our natural immune system and our defense mechanisms which protect us against any germs or other aggressors.

■ It calms an overactive mind.

■ It stimulates and lifts depression.

■ It restores our feelings of self worth, happiness and contentment.

■ It restores concentration and alertness.

■ It increases our general state of well-being.

■ It strengthens our self-confidence and provides us with the necessary will power to face our daily problems with confidence and happiness.

with one another; it can be a fascinating journey to imagine how all the cells in our body work together simultaneously and in synchronistic rhythm.

Life is a balance between tension and relaxation, between a state of balance or harmony and a state of imbalance or disharmony, a charge and discharge of energy in its purest forms. Our bodies, through our aches and pains, let us know when this balance has been disturbed or, in some severe circumstances, destroyed. The causes may be either emotional problems or environmental influences which destroy the flow of energy and as a result we feel drained, washed out, lacking in strength and generally unwell. It is when we find ourselves with any of these imbalances that an aromatherapy massage can help us to access and restore the normal and healthy synchronicity between all the cells in the body.

PREPARING FOR MASSAGE

1 Ensure that the room is warm and well ventilated.

2 Check that the working area, either a special massage couch or the floor, is well covered with some warm towels and that there are sufficient towels, blankets and pillows to make the treatment enjoyable for the giver and the receiver.

3 Choose a room where the lights can be dimmed and soft music can be played.

4 Make sure that there will be no interruptions during the period of time when the massage is carried out. For example, switch off the phone ringer, or if you have children ask a friend to look after them for you.

5 When attempting self-massage or giving massage to a receiver, you should wear loose and comfortable clothing, for if you, as the giver, are uncomfortable this will be perceived by your recipient and will disrupt the flow and rhythm of the massage.

6 Prior to giving a massage, your nails should be cut short, so as not to hurt your partner's skin.

7 Your hands should always be clean, washed and, if cold, warmed by rubbing them together. Never give a massage with cold hands; it will create tension instead of relaxation in the receiver.

8 Prepare your massage oil by blending your essential oils in your chosen carrier oil in a proportion of three percent of essential oils and 97 percent of a carrier or vegetable oil.

9 Have a cup of herbal tea, such as Chamomile or Rosehip, ready for your partner to drink prior to the massage to initiate the detoxifying process which will be encouraged by the massage.

10 Depending on the area of the body to be massaged, you should ask the receiver to remove her/his clothes either in part or completely. In the latter case, you should have a robe ready for him/her to wear.

11 While giving a massage, try to maintain contact with the receiver's body at all times. If you have to move around, keep one hand in contact with his/her body to ensure their feeling of confidence.

MASSAGE MOVEMENTS

The following massage movements are always repeated and hence you should be familiar with their terminology and therapeutic effects.

STROKING OR EFFLEURAGE

In this movement you glide with your hands lying flat over the receiver's body, stroking with light pressure over the areas to be worked on, and contouring the body. This movement always commences and ends any sequence. You should work from the periphery to the center, always in the direction of the heart, to guide all body fluids in the direction of the circulation.

Effleurage movements help to mobilize the lymph and diminish the localized pockets of accumulated fluid which may later cause imbalances and disruptions.

Below: effleurage is a stroking movement, molding the body.

They also stimulate the nerve endings which are distributed all over the surface of the body, waking up all areas.

KNEADING OR PETRISSAGE

This movement is carried out by lifting the skin and muscle tissue between the thumb and fingers of each hand in turn and carrying out a kneading movement, similar to that of kneading dough to make bread, then smoothing the tissue out gently. Each hand works in sequence with the other: while one squeezes, the other relaxes until the whole area worked on is covered.

Kneading improves the muscle's tone and circulation, helps to alleviate tension and, when carried out vigorously, enhances muscle metabolism and prevents the accumulation of toxins.

Below: when kneading, the hands squeeze and relax in sequence.

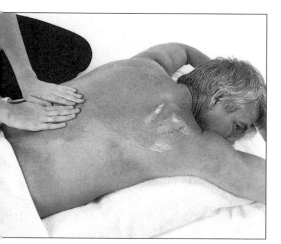

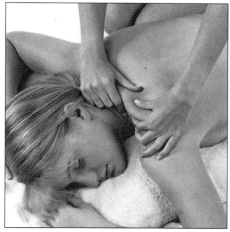

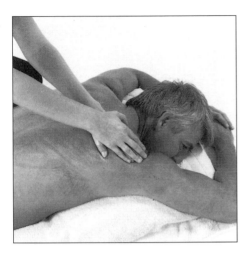

Above: pressures are applied at regular intervals on the body.

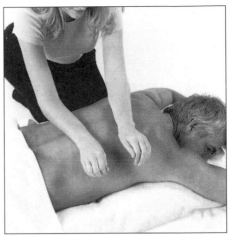

Above: cupping is a stimulating stroke sometimes used in aromatherapy massage.

PRESSURES

These movements are carried out by applying pressures at regular intervals along the various pressure points located on the face, spine, and limbs, corresponding to acupuncture meridians. This technique increases the blood supply to the tissues and increases cell renewal. The movements are also very beneficial for pain relief due to their direct effect on the peripheral nerve endings and their transmission to the central nervous system.

TAPOTEMENT

These movements include hacking, cupping, plucking, pummeling and other percussion techniques, which are very stimulating. However, they are very rarely an integral part of the aromatherapy massage treatment.

PREPARATION OF THE TREATMENT BLEND

A blend is the name given to the massage oil formulation which consists of one essential oil, or several essential oils and a single carrier oil, or various carrier oils mixed together. A good tip is to separately prepare your blend or mix of essential oils and that of your carrier oils.

1 If you choose three essential oils, prepare a blend which contains either equal parts of all three or a larger amount of the one you need or like the most. Place the essential oils in a 5ml amber glass bottle and roll the bottle gently between your palms to mix the oils.

2 Tip the bottle, holding it by its top and base with your index finger and thumb, three times. This will ensure a thorough molecular blend of essential oils.

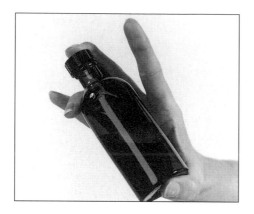

Above: to mix the essential and carrier oils, roll and tip the bottle.

3 Decide whether you would like to use just one carrier oil or if you would like to add some other carrier oils for their nourishing and anti-ageing effects. For instance, in a 50ml amber glass bottle you may like to use 30ml of Sweet Almond oil as your base and add to it 10ml of Rosehip oil and 10ml of Avocado oil, thus having a total of 50ml as your base oil.

4 The next step is to add your essential oil to your carrier oils; the most frequently used proportion is three percent. Therefore to 48.5ml of carrier oil you add 1.5ml of your prepared blend of essential oils. The easiest way of achieving this is to decant 1.5ml of carrier oil from your 50ml and then add the essential oils. Use the same palm rolling and tipping procedure to ensure a thorough and even blend.

This 50ml of your prepared massage oil should be sufficient for between four and five full body treatments, depending on the type of skin and size of the recipient.

AROMATHERAPY MASSAGE SEQUENCE

My preferred aromatherapy massage sequence begins by massaging the back, followed by the back of the lower limbs, including the feet. Then I ask the receiver to turn around and I continue the massage, beginning with the front of the feet and ascending along the lower limbs, then the abdomen, the chest and the upper limbs, ending with the head, neck, and face.

I choose to finish with the face, as I find that this concludes the treatment in a very relaxing and enjoyable manner. By this time the recipient is almost asleep and is able to luxuriate and unwind completely, if only for a few minutes. Once the massage has ended, I find it beneficial to leave him/her resting for five to 10 minutes before waking them up with a glass of water or a cup of herbal tea, helping them to sit up and allowing them to get dressed.

BACK MASSAGE

The receiver should be lying face down on the couch with a supporting pillow or a rolled towel under the ankles and, if necessary, under the breasts. Before uncovering the back, make contact through the towel and stretch the back by placing your forearms in the center and smoothing them out in opposite directions toward the head and the lower back. Then uncover the back gently, leaving the towel and covering blanket at the level of the lower back or the upper thigh.

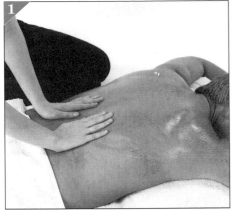

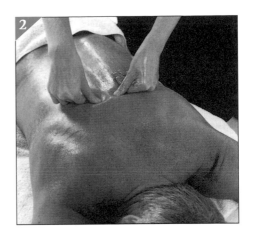

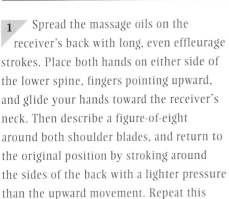

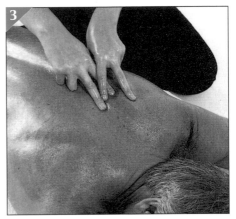

1   Spread the massage oils on the receiver's back with long, even effleurage strokes. Place both hands on either side of the lower spine, fingers pointing upward, and glide your hands toward the receiver's neck. Then describe a figure-of-eight around both shoulder blades, and return to the original position by stroking around the sides of the back with a lighter pressure than the upward movement. Repeat this stroke three times.

2   Place one hand next to the other on the right-hand side of the receiver's spine and, with both thumbs, glide in. Press gently for a few seconds and glide upward into each intervertebral space, until you reach the cervical spine, then glide down to your initial position. Repeat three times on each side of the spine. With both hands on the right-hand side of the spine describe gliding and fanning toward and upward with stroking movements until you reach the shoulder blade (scapula). Then glide down to your initial position. Repeat three times on each side.

3   Glide your hands to the top of the spine, and position the index and middle fingers of your right hand astride the sides of the spine. Do the same with the index and middle fingers of your left hand and position them above the fingers of your right hand, then glide down the sides of the spine, positioning each hand alternately in front of the other. This gives the sensation of a continuous downward stroking movement and is very soothing and relaxing. Glide to the start and repeat three times.

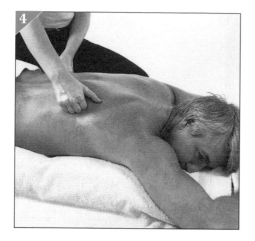

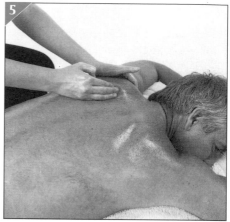

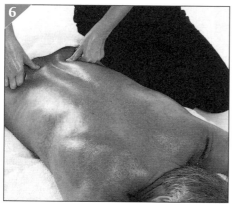

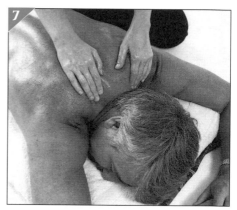

4 Beginning at the lower back, knead the right-hand side of the receiver's body, moving toward the shoulder, then with smaller kneading movements repeat the sequence commencing at the bottom. Always remember to glide downward. Repeat three times on each side. Glide to the buttocks and then knead each buttock thoroughly.

5 Place the hands over the sacrum (center lower back) and press with your thumbs, outlining the sacrum. Repeat this movement three times.

6 Glide up to the right shoulder, cup the shoulder with one hand and, with the edge of the other hand, outline the inner edge of the shoulder blade three times. If you find any tight areas, try smoothing them out with your thumbs. Repeat the same on the other side.

7 Place your hands, cupping the nape of the neck on either side of the spine, and with your fingers gently describe small circles on either side of the neck. Finish the back massage with a long, light effleurage stroke all over the back.

BACK OF THE LEGS MASSAGE

1 Lift the foot and work around the inner and outer ankle bones with circular movements, which help to relax and stimulate at the same time.

2 Place the foot on the couch or floor and place both hands around the leg, with both thumbs facing the center of the calf, slightly pressing. Glide upward toward the back of the knee, and then release the pressure about one inch below the knee fold.

3 Continue gliding without pressure up one inch above the fold, then repeat the previous pressure in an upward sweeping movement until you reach the fold between the thighs and the buttocks.

4 Stop with your inner hand at the fold, and with your outer hand sweep inward. This movement guides the lymph towards the lymph nodes of the groin and helps to shift any accumulated toxins. Glide down and repeat three times. Knead the thigh from the knee to the buttock, dividing it into two sections: outer and inner. In people with very heavy thighs you may divide them into three sections for the purpose of kneading. Repeat three times. Continue in the same way with the left leg.

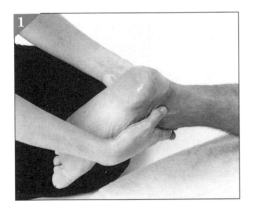

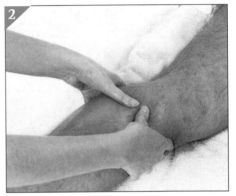

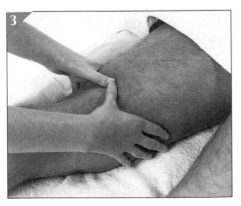

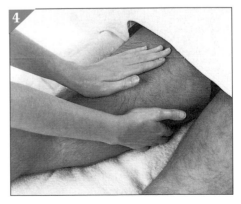

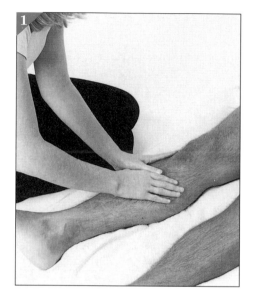

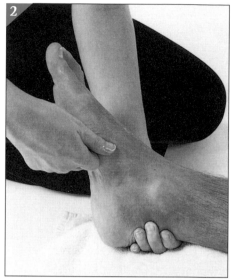

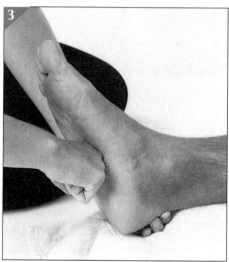

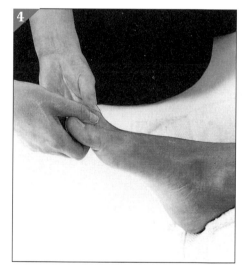

FRONT OF THE LOWER LIMBS

1 Uncover the right lower limb (leg). Spread the oil blend on the whole area ready for the massage.

2 Lift the foot by holding the ankle with your left hand. Then, with your right hand, pinch along the inner edge

of the foot from the toes to the heel.

3 With your hand in a fist, work on the hollow of the foot in a circular manner to smooth out any tight areas.

4 Commencing with the large toe, work gently on each of the joints of each toe in a circular motion.

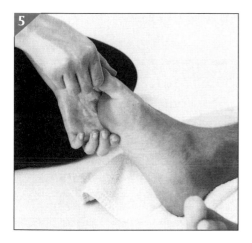

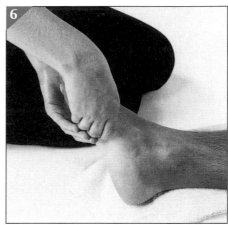

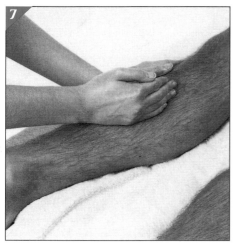

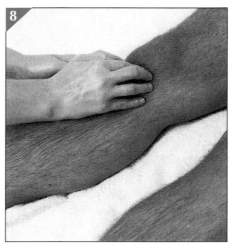

5 Then hold each toe between your index and middle fingers and pull outward toward the tip of the toe, shaking out your hands after each toe to pull out any "energies" which may be stagnated there.

6 Hold the ball of the foot with both hands and lightly pull forward to open up the foot and improve the circulation.

7 Hold the shin with one hand, and with the other make a slicing downward movement next to the shin bone from the knee to the ankle. Repeat on the inner side of the bone. This movement helps to strengthen the muscle fibers which are attached to this bone.

8 Glide up to the knee cap and, with both hands, make circular movements defining the edge of the knee cap. This will encourage the blood and lymph circulation and avoid the formation of pockets of fluid under the knee cap.

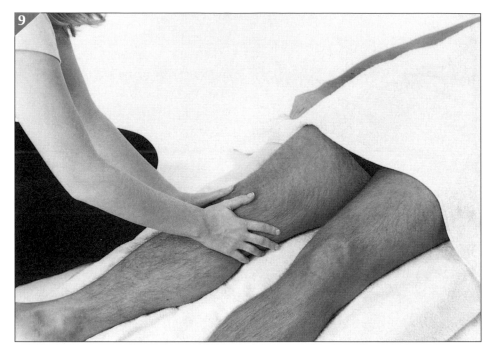

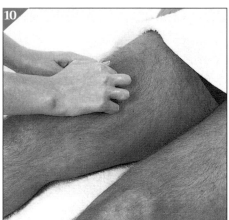

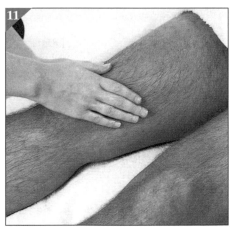

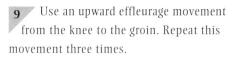

9 Use an upward effleurage movement from the knee to the groin. Repeat this movement three times.

10 Knead the front of the thighs in the same way as you did with the back of the thighs. Always end any movement

with an inward sweep at the groin.

11 Glide to the ankle and finish the front of the leg with a long, sweeping effleurage movement from the ankle to the groin. Cover the right leg with a towel. Uncover the left leg and repeat the sequence.

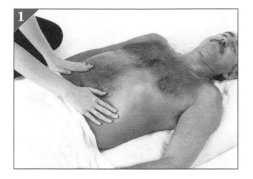

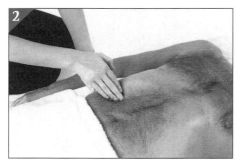

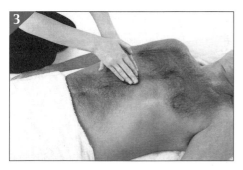

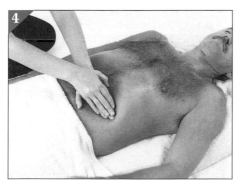

THE ABDOMEN

Before embarking on an abdominal massage always remember that this is the most vulnerable part of the receiver's body. It is not protected by bones and contains the internal organs of digestion. The lower part, or pelvis, contains the urinary and reproductive organs, and the upper part also contains a large number of nerve endings and nerve groups called plexus, the main one being the solar plexus which is traditionally known as the center of our emotions.

1 Begin the massage of the abdomen by gently spreading the massage oil all over the surface and, with light pressure, outline a diamond shape naturally formed by the lower part of the rib cage at the top and the pelvic bones at the bottom.

2 Place one hand over the other and, beginning at the right side of your partner's abdomen, work upward from the pelvis to the rib cage.

3 Then work across to the left side of the rib cage and, lastly, downward to the left of the pelvic bone.

4 This should be done in a circular clockwise even stroke. Repeat three times, always decreasing the pressure when passing from left to right. This is because you are working around the colon or large intestine and it finishes with the rectum and anus on the bottom left-hand side when it is deeper. If you work anticlockwise this would alter the natural peristaltic contractions (normal bowel movements) and may produce nausea.

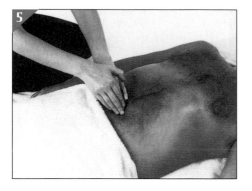

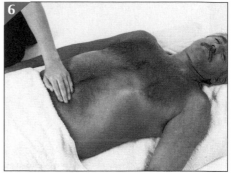

5 Repeat the same circular movement, describing a smaller circle inside the area previously covered. Repeat three times. Place both hands on the navel and work in a star shape, gliding from the navel upward toward the sternum and back, then to the right and back, to the left and back, and finally downward and back to the navel. Repeat the star shape three times.

6 Place your hand, cupping the navel, and leave it there for a couple of minutes to restore the balance and centering. Cover the abdomen with a towel.

CHEST MASSAGE

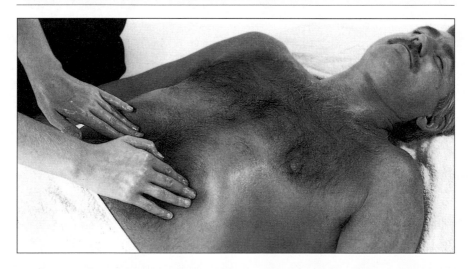

Never work on the breasts. The chest massage is restricted to outlining the edges of the ribs on either side between the fingers and thumb to stimulate the lymph drainage.

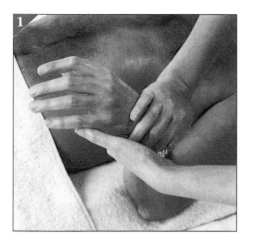

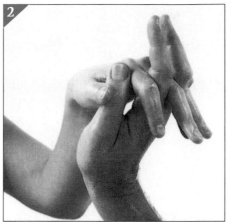

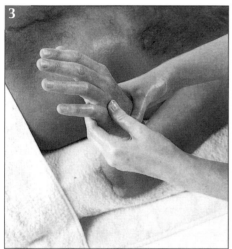

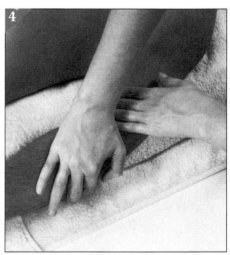

THE UPPER LIMBS

1 Uncover the right upper limb (arm) and commence the massage by massaging the hand in the following manner. Spread the massage oil blend evenly on the palm and the upper side of the receiver's hand.

2 Now open the receiver's hand by interlocking your fingers with their fingers and gently stretching. Repeat twice.

3 Work on the joints of each finger in the same way as you did with the toes.

4 Work your way upward to the wrist with long effleurage movements, then work up the forearm until you reach the arm and armpit with long, soothing movements, increasing the pressure each time you repeat the movement. Repeat three times and finish at the armpit. Repeat with the other upper limb.

FACIAL AROMATHERAPY

An aromatherapy facial is a very relaxing and, at the same time, an uplifting experience. Find a quiet place in your home, pull the drapes or lower the blinds, switch off the phone and ensure that you have between 15 and 30 minutes to yourself. Put on your favorite music and cleanse your face gently with some aromatic cleansing milk.

AROMA-ENERGY FACIAL

Overleaf you will find a step-by-step illustrated aroma-energy facial massage, which aims to increase or decrease energy, which can cause anxiety and tension. When you are feeling particularly tired or tense, perhaps after a busy day, you could make some quiet time to try this massage to help invigorate and relax you.

All movements are carried out to either increase (concentrate) or decrease (disperse) energy. The movements are made with the forefingers of both hands working symmetrically and simultaneously on the face.

All movements are light and spiraling, and the pressure on the facial skin is almost imperceptible. In fact, the pressure utilized in this sequence has been poetically compared to the pressure required to hold a butterfly's wings in between the surface of the face and that of the fingertips—sufficient to hold, yet not enough to cause any damage to the butterfly.

When the need is to concentrate energy on focal points the fingers spiral inward, whereas where it is considered necessary to release or decrease energy, the spiraling movements go in an outward motion so as to remove excessive energy which is the cause of tension and anxiety.

The movements are performed sequentially with the fingers lifted after each point massaged with this technique.

THE ADVANTAGES OF THIS TECHNIQUE

The beauty of this aroma-energy facial technique is that you can perform it on yourself, either sitting up or lying down comfortably with your head supported by pillows. Alternatively, you can do it with your partner, or use it to relax your nearest and dearest child. It is a wonderful effort-free way of removing all worries, fear, and strain.

An aroma-energy facial can help promote parent-child bonding, enhance your relationship and mutual understanding with your partner, and aid self-relaxation. It is an ideal relaxation technique when you have only a quarter of an hour to relax and to forget all the tensions, worries, and anticipation experienced before an important meeting or interview.

Unlike many relaxation and aromatherapy massage techniques, it can be carried out anywhere, at any time and requires nothing more than a few drops of your favorite blend. It is thoroughly recommended by everyone who has benefited from this technique.

SIMPLE FACIAL

1 Commencing in the middle of your forehead, stroke gently with both your thumbs toward your temples. Repeat this three times.

2 With your middle and index fingers, draw spirals with your fingertips, moving from the center toward your temples in six steps, finishing with some gentle pressure on the temples.

3 Walk your fingers down the sides of your nose, alternating on both sides. Walk your fingers from the center of the area above your upper lip to your temples. Draw spirals from your chin to your temples, from the corners of your mouth to your temples, and from the sides of your nose to your temples.

4 Press the palms of both hands on your face, covering the area between your chin and earlobes, then sweep down your throat and outward across your collar bones to your armpits.

Note: you should ensure that your fingers are completely relaxed and the massage movements come from your arms. The massage should be in time with your pulse in a rhythmic manner.

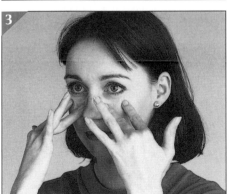

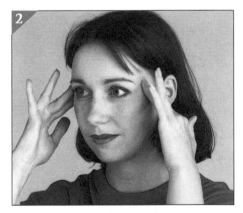

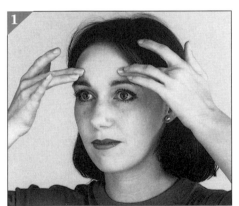

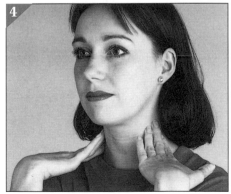

AROMA-ENERGY FACIAL

Remember that in this massage all the movements are performed in the sequence shown here. When you have massaged each individual focal point, as per the instructions below, lift your fingers and then move on to the next point that is indicated. There are 12 pressure points in total.

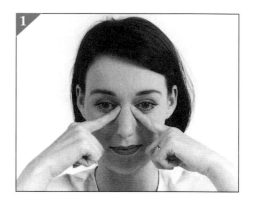

1 Start the aroma-energy facial massage by working on the five points located around each eye. Commence by pressing lightly on the inner corner of the eye, then lift your fingers and move on to the next point.

2 Now place your index fingers on the innermost point of the eyebrows, pressing lightly.

3 Remove your fingers and reposition them in the center of each eyebrow. Remember to keep the pressure almost imperceptible.

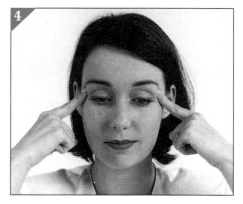

4 Now place each index finger at the outer corner of each eye.

5 Move on to the last of the five points around the eyes, and press on the center of the bony ridge below the lower eyelids.

6 Working in the same manner, move on to the four pressure points which are located around the cheekbones. Start by pressing on the point located on the side of the lower third of the nose.

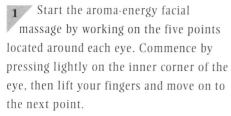

7 Now move down the cheekbone and press on the center of the ridge under each cheekbone.

8 Next press with your index fingers on the outer edge of each cheekbone, near the earlobes.

9 For the last point in this cheekbone sequence, press on the point that is located between points 6 and 8, as shown.

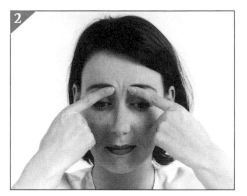

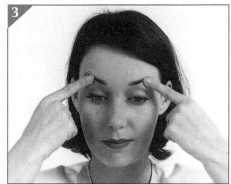

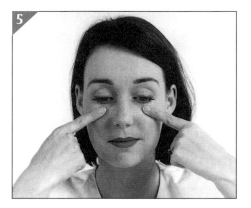

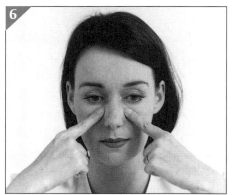

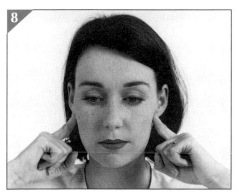

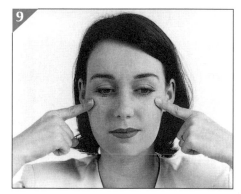

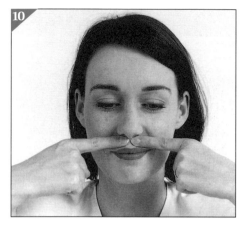

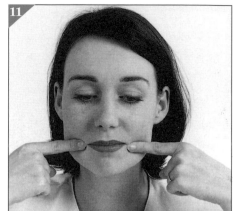

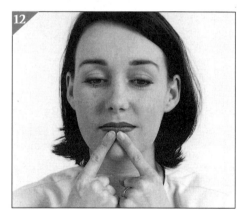

10 The last sequence is carried out on three pressure points around the mouth. The first one is in the center of the area above the upper lip.

11 This is followed by placing one finger on each corner of the mouth and then working simultaneously and symmetrically on the outer corners.

12 Finally, press lightly on the last pressure point in the center of the area below the lower lip.

FACIAL MASSAGE OILS

This simple sequence of 12 specific light pressure points provides a very effective relaxing and energizing massage, which is easy to perform and eases headaches, tiredness, and insomnia.

Because of the type of massage, only the most exquisite essential oils, such as Rose and Neroli should be utilized, diluted as a one percent dilution of Camellia and Jojoba oils in almost equal proportions, e.g. one drop of Neroli with 49 drops of Camellia and 50 drops of Jojoba (total of 100 drops/5ml).

The basic massage sequence described above may be adapted to the needs of the recipient by focusing on the massage of the back, the face, the hands etc. and not giving a full body massage, or by performing only light effleurage movements if your partner is not sure that a deeper massage is a good idea. More specific variations are described in further chapters.

NECK MASSAGE

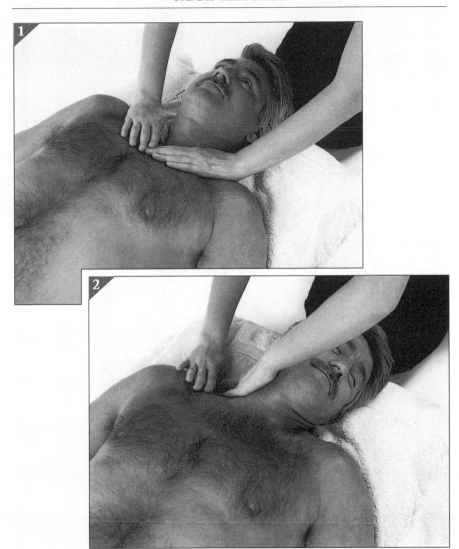

1 Work your way up to the neck, pressing around the edges of the collar bone from the sternum or center to the shoulders. Repeat the massage movement three times.

2 Turn your partner's head to the left and gently work from the jaw downward to the shoulder, describing three downward draining lines. Repeat both the above movements on the opposite side.

CHAPTER FOUR

AROMATHERAPY FOR ENERGY & RELAXATION

Aromatherapy provides an ideal form of treatment for those times when you are feeling jaded, low, and lacking the energy that is needed to finish those urgently required jobs. Or it can be beneficial on those occasions when you have come home after a long day at work, or have had a very busy and tiring day with your young children and need to summon up some extra energy to be able to change and get ready for that unexpected special occasion.

A full body massage with special emphasis on the stimulating and energizing movements described below, is one of the most effective ways of recharging your batteries and restoring much needed balance.

REVITALIZING MASSAGE

Invigorating movements, such as kneading and wringing, use squeezing and rolling to increase the blood supply to the muscles and thus make them warmer and more pliable. Invigorating kneading movements can be performed on tense shoulders, the lower back, and aching limbs to revitalize and re-energize them.

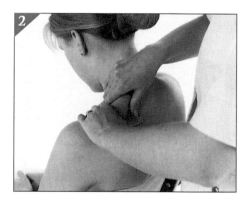

1 Stand behind your partner. Place both hands on the left shoulder. Press down with one hand to gather and lift the trapezius muscle and the flesh underneath it between your fingers and thumb. Roll and release it into your other hand.

Continue doing this for three to five minutes, then repeat the movement on the right shoulder.

2 If the shoulders are very tight, press even deeper with your fingers, and incorporate a slight twisting movement.

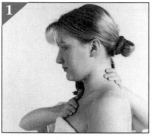
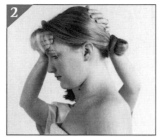
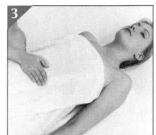
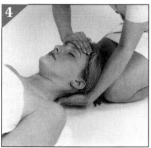
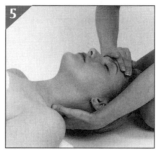
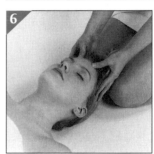

FOR RELIEVING TENSION

1 Standing, place one hand on the center of the receiver's chest with the palm of your other hand at the same level on her back. Ask the receiver to breathe deeply while you glide both hands upward until you reach the shoulders.

2 Keeping your hand on the back of the neck, slowly move to the crown at the top of the skull, with your other hand on the receiver's forehead. Ask them to imagine their tension and worries floating away and that energy and vitality are flowing into their system.

3 To re-energize the lower back, place your nearest hand under the lower back, and ask the receiver to drop her back into your hand. With your other hand above the lower belly, ask them to deepen and slow their breathing and relax into your hands. Gently describe some small circular movements with the hand which is supporting the lower back.

4 To re-energize stiff and painful head, neck, and shoulder areas, place the receiver's head in your cupped left hand, while your right hand rests on their forehead.

5 Slowly press with your fingertips into the muscle at the base of the skull and feel the bony ridge. Make tiny circular movements on one spot at a time, working gradually toward the spine and finishing where the cervical spine joins the skull. Roll the receiver's head into your right hand and repeat the movement twice.

6 With both hands, gently bring the head back into alignment with the spine and move your hands onto the chest to glide over the sternum or breastbone, outward over the shoulders, and up to the tip of the hair above the head.

ENERGIZING ESSENTIAL OILS

These additional energizing sequences add those special extra touches to the basic massage outline described in Chapter Three. The main essential oils that are recommended for their use in revitalizing and energizing formulations are: Bergamot, Ginger, Spike Lavender, Lemon, Neroli, Scots Pine, Petitgrain, Rosemary, Rose, Rosewood and Sandalwood.

ENERGIZING FORMULATIONS

The following formulations have proven extremely beneficial for revitalizing and energizing treatments of people suffering from tiredness and lethargy.

MASSAGE FORMULATION 1

Essential oil of Lemon	
(Citrus limonum):	2 drops
Essential oil of Scots Pine	
(Pinus sylvestris):	2 drops
Essential oil of Rosemary	
(Rosmarinus officinalis):	2 drops
Wheatgerm base oil:	14 drops
Sweet Almond base oil:	9ml
Total amount:	**10ml**

Note: in all massage formulations the maximum proportion of essential oils should be three percent.

MASSAGE FORMULATION 2

Essential oil of Cypress	
(Cupressus sempervirens):	4 drops
Essential oil of Bergamot	
(Citrus bergamia):	3 drops
Essential oil of Ginger	
(Zingiber officinalis):	2 drops
Essential oil of Orange	
(Citrus aurantium ssp amara):	2 drops
Essential oil of Vetiver	
(Vetiveria zizanoides):	1 drop
Rosehip seed base oil	
(Rosa rubiginosa):	4 ml
Apricot kernel base oil:	15.5ml
Total amount:	**20ml**

BATH FORMULATION 1

Essential oil of Scots Pine	
(Pinus sylvestris):	2 drops
Essential oil of Sandalwood	
(Santalum album):	2 drops
Essential oil of Rosemary	
(Rosmarinus officinalis):	1 drop
Dispersing bath oil:	1 teaspoon

BATH FORMULATION 2

Essential oil of Neroli	
(Citrus aurantium ssp amara):	1 drop
Essential oil of Petitgrain	
(Citrus aurantium ssp amara):	2 drops
Essential oil of Orange	
(Citrus aurantium ssp amara):	2 drops
Dispersing bath oil:	1 teaspoon

AROMATHERAPY FOR RELAXATION

Aromatherapy is a very effective form of treatment for stress, helping to prevent any damage arising from constant stress and tension. It can also be beneficial when stress is already giving rise to other symptoms, such as irritability, tiredness, insomnia, and backache.

An aromatherapy treatment creates a relaxing and calming atmosphere, whether in the form of a massage, the addition of three to five drops of your favorite essential oil or blend of oils to a morning or evening bath, or the burning and vaporizing of essential oils such as Bergamot, Sandalwood, Vetiver or Ylang Ylang. In this atmosphere tension is diffused, tranquillity flows and our inner physical, mental, emotional, and spiritual core is touched.

Many stress-related problems, such as headaches, backache, stomach butterflies, and indigestion will benefit and respond well to aromatherapy treatments.

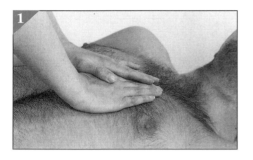

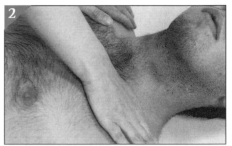

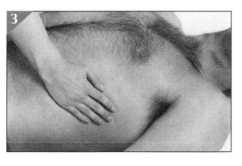

RELAXING MASSAGE MOVEMENTS

To relax and calm the receiver's body you can use certain specific smooth, flowing, effleurage strokes which enhance physical and psychological well-being. The following movements will help to relax them.

1 With the receiver lying on his/her back, stand at their side and position your hands at the base of the sternum or breast bone, with your fingers pointing upward toward the receiver's chin.

2 Glide both hands upward and describe a fanning movement outward toward the receiver's shoulders, then let your hands envelope the shoulders, and slide down around the armpits to the sides of the body.

3 Molding your hands to the shape of the body, slide along the edge of the rib cage with slightly more pressure. Repeat several times to induce a deeply relaxing effect on the receiver.

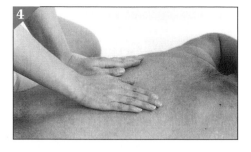

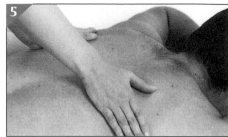

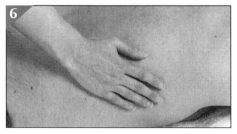

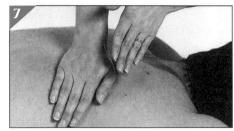

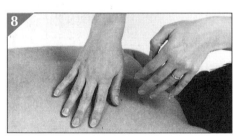

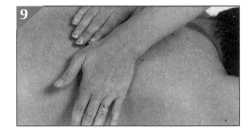

4 With the receiver lying face-down, describe small fan-shaped slow strokes on their back; these are relaxing and restful, but, if performed more rapidly, they are refreshing.

5 Place the flat of your hands on the receiver's skin and glide up steadily, then, after a short distance, fan out to the sides.

6 Glide back down the body and softly mold it with your hands. Lightly get back to the beginning and repeat several times, each time beginning at a higher point of the receiver's back. Then with your fingers pointing downward, stroke slowly with the flat of one hand following the other. Lift

one hand slowly while the other takes its place very gently.

7 Repeat by returning the first hand to the body and lifting the second hand.

8 This should be perceived as a slow, continuous movement by the receiver to soothe the nervous system and settle down and relax their body.

9 Another gentle movement is known as feather stroking in which your fingers should only touch the skin very lightly in a downward flowing movement. This movement is very relaxing, not only on the back but also on the limbs.

RELAXING ESSENTIAL OILS

The following formulations have proven very beneficial for aromatherapy relaxation treatments of people who are suffering from tension, stress, and anxiety.

MASSAGE FORMULATION 1

Essential oil of Bergamot	
(Citrus aurantium bergamia):	2 drops
Essential oil of Sandalwood	
(Santalum album):	2 drops
Essential oil of Rosewood	
(Aniba rosaeodora var *amazonica):*	2 drops
Wheatgerm base oil:	14 drops
Sweet Almond base oil:	9ml
Total amount:	**10ml**

MASSAGE FORMULATION 2

Essential oil of Roman Chamomile	
(Anthemis nobilis):	2 drops
Essential oil of Petitgrain	
(Citrus aurantium ssp aurantium):	3 drops
Essential oil of Fine Lavender	
(Lavandula angustifolia):	3 drops
Essential oil of Bergamot	
(Citrus aurantium ssp bergamia):	2 drops
Essential oil of Orange	
(Citrus aurantium ssp aurantium):	2 drops
Rosehip seed base oil	
(Rosa rubiginosa):	4ml
Apricot kernel base oil:	15.5ml
Total amount:	**20ml**

Note: in all massage formulations the maximum proportion of essential oils should be three percent.

BATH FORMULATION 1

Essential oil of Fine Lavender	
(Lavandula angustifolia):	2 drops
Essential oil of Sandalwood	
(Santalum album):	2 drops
Essential oil of Roman Chamomile	
(Anthemis nobilis):	1 drop
Dispersing bath oil:	1 teaspoon

BATH FORMULATION 2

Essential oil of Neroli	
(Citrus aurantium ssp amara):	1 drop
Essential oil of Petitgrain	
(Citrus aurantium ssp amara):	2 drops
Essential oil of Geranium	
(Pelargonium odorantissimum):	2 drops
Dispersing bath oil:	1 teaspoon

BATH FORMULATION 3

Essential oil of Roman Chamomile	
(Anthemis nobilis):	2 drops
Essential oil of Fine Lavender	
(Lavandula angustifolia):	2 drops
Essential oil of Lavandin	
(Lavandula hybrida):	1 drop
Dispersing bath oil:	1 teaspoon

Note: the above amounts are calculated to be sufficient for a bath in a full bath tub. It is better to mix them immediately before going into the water as explained in Chapter Three (see page 69).

CHAPTER FIVE

HEALTH TREATMENTS & BEAUTY

All essential oils have powerful healing properties which may help in the prevention and treatment of diseases and imbalances that affect our physical, mental, emotional, and spiritual well-being. Essential oils are very beneficial for self-help treatments for many minor ailments before calling your doctor.

TREATING STRESS-RELATED COMPLAINTS

The prolonged and persistent pressures of daily life and work may lead to a variety of gradually worsening symptoms which are felt by the sufferer including the following.

■ Insomnia

This is sleeplessness from overtiredness, with a great difficulty in unwinding, relaxing and achieving a restful night's sleep. You feel unable to go to sleep and the next day you are very irritable, tired, and unable to carry out your work.

Aromatherapy offers many ways of helping this problem. You may wish to:

1 Place one or two drops of an essential oil with relaxing properties, e.g. Fine Lavender (*Lavandula angustifolia*), Roman Chamomile (*Anthemis nobilis*), Neroli (*Citrus aurantium ssp amara*), or Rosewood (*Aniba rosaeodora* var *amazonica*) on your pillow.

2 Take a comforting evening bath with any of the relaxing oils before going to bed.

3 Ask your partner to give you a relaxing massage with your favorite blend of essential oils in a base oil.

All of the above methods are known to help greatly with insomnia. The advantage of using these treatments instead of medication is that you wake up refreshed, and not with a fuzzy head. They also offer a very pleasant alternative to medication.

■ Benign hypertension

This is a mild rise in the blood pressure due to an emotional upset or over-work. At this stage it may be a better idea to try aromatherapy rather than conventional medication with diuretics or beta blockers. Before you try these treatments get your doctor's agreement.

1 Aromatic baths with either of the following formulations:

Essential oil of Roman Chamomile (*Anthemis nobilis*):	2 drops
Essential oil of Petitgrain (*Citrus aurantium ssp amara*):	1 drop
Essential oil of Fine Lavender (*Lavandula angustifolia*):	2 drops
Sweet Almond oil:	1 teaspoon

2 Or ask your partner to give you a relaxing massage with:

Essential oil of Sandalwood
(Santalum album): 2 drops
Essential oil of Marjoram
(Origanum majorana): 3 drops
Essential oil of Geranium
(Pelargonium odorantissimum): 3 drops
Rosehip seed oil *(Rosa rubiginosa):* 4.5ml
Apricot kernel oil: 10ml
Total amount of formulation: 15ml

■ Mental fatigue or nervous exhaustion

When you feel unable to get out of bed and face the world for no apparent reason, or you feel you lack the confidence to get on with your life, a regular aromatherapy treatment may help you to return to an even keel.

1 An aromatic bath with your favorite blend of stimulating and energizing oils may help you to face the day.

2 An aromatherapy massage with the revitalizing oils and techniques described may be just what you need.

MINOR ACCIDENTS

In those minor accidents in the home, when first aid is required, the following is recommended:

■ Children's bumps and bruises

It is always recommended to have Spike Lavender (*Lavandula latifolia*) and Fine Lavender (*Lavandula angustifolia*) in the first aid box. Two to three drops of either on a cold handkerchief or some lint placed over the bruise will speed up the healing process. Depending on the severity it may heal in a few hours or a few days. In the

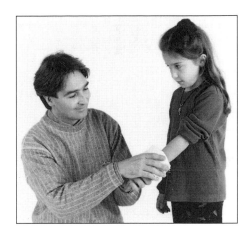

Above: a cold Lavender compress will help to heal bruises.

latter case, the compress should be replaced and renewed every 12 hours. A practical tip is to wrap some plastic wrap around the compress to avoid getting wet clothes.

■ Minor burns

For those burns caused by accidentally touching a hot iron or a hot oven tray, two or three drops of Spike Lavender (*Lavandula latifolia*) will encourage the healing process and avoid blistering. Repeat this application three to four times a day as required. Please make sure that only the recommended drops are used undiluted on the skin.

■ Childhood diseases

Once the disease has been diagnosed by your doctor, it is very helpful to bathe your child in the following formulation of anti-infectious essential oils:
Essential oil of Eucalyptus R.
(Eucalyptus radiata): 1 drop

Essential oil of Tea Tree
(Melaleuca alternifolia): 1 drop
Essential oil of Fine Lavender
(Lavandula angustifolia): 2 drops
Essential oil of Roman Chamomile
(Anthemis nobilis): 2 drops
Turkish red dispersing bath oil: 1 teaspoon

With the recommended aromatherapy bath technique described in Chapter 3 (see page 69), twice daily prepare your child's bath with:
One quarter of the prepared formulation for a child aged one to four years;
Half of the prepared formulation twice daily for four to eight-year-old children;
The whole amount for children aged eight years and over.

This treatment should be followed for a period of seven days. This formulation helps to keep the child's temperature normal, guards against secondary infections, and helps the child to feel relaxed and contented despite being covered in a rash.

■ Coughs and colds

Aromatherapy inhalations are ideal for the treatment of upper respiratory tract infections. The following essential oils should be used following the technique described in Chapter Three (see page 70).
Adults: Tea Tree *(Melaleuca alternifolia)*, Eucalyptus Globulus or Eucalyptus Radiata, Sandalwood *(Santalum album)*, Manuka *(Leptospermum scoparium)*.
Young children: Tea Tree *(Melaleuca alternifolia)*, Sandalwood *(Santalum album)*,

Frankincense *(Boswellia carterii)*, Lemon *(Citrus limonum)*. Use inhalation oils in a diffuser as young children may have difficulty inhaling.

A massage formulation may be prepared for younger children with three drops made up of two to three of the above listed essential oils in 10ml of Apricot kernel base oil.

■ Premenstrual tension

To relieve tension and fluid retention in those few days prior to a menstrual period the following formulation may be used added to the water in the bath:
Essential oil of Cypress
(Cupressus sempervirens): 2 drops
Essential oil of Moroccan Chamomile
(Ormenis mixta): 2 drops
Essential oil of Geranium
(Pelargonium odorantissimum): 3 drops
Essential oil of Marjoram
(Origanum majorana): 3 drops
Rosehip seed base oil: 4ml
Evening Primrose base oil: 4ml
Sweet Almond base oil: 6.5ml
Total amount of formulation: 15ml
Note: use 10 drops of this preparation daily in your evening bath. Alternatively, massage your lower back and abdomen with a small amount of the blend daily for a period no longer than seven days.

■ Diarrhea and constipation

When these symptoms are due to mild food poisoning, and there is no detection of a gram negative pathogen by the doctor and pathology laboratory, use the following formulation in massage of the lower abdomen:

Essential oil of Ajowan
(Tachispermum anni):   1 drop

Essential oil of Roman Chamomile
(Anthemis nobilis):   5 drops

Essential oil of Ginger
(Zingiber officinalis):   4 drops

Essential oil of Lemon
(Citrus limonum):   4 drops

Sweet Almond base oil: 20.5 ml

Total amount of formulation: **21 ml**

Massage the lower back and abdomen two or three times daily until cramps and pain cease.

■ Acne

This skin condition is usually due to a hormonal imbalance in the pubertal years. An effective topical aromatherapy formulation is the following:

Essential oil of Fine Lavender
(Lavandula angustifolia):   6 drops

Essential oil of Spike Lavender
(Lavandula latifolia):   6 drops

Essential oil of Lavandin
(Lavandula hybrida):   6 drops

Essential oil of Sandalwood
(Santalum album):   6 drops

Base may be either distilled
water or Aloe Vera gel   30 gr.

Apply the lotion to the affected areas after cleansing with a gentle, non-alcoholic cleansing lotion.

■ Mouth ulcers

These are infectious ulcers in the mouth, inside the cheeks, or gums, which are aggravated by acid foods. They respond very well to aromatherapy. Topical, direct application of essential oils of Tea Tree *(Melaleuca alternifolia)*, Cypress *(Cupressus sempervirens)* or Lemon *(Citrus limonum)*, as well as mouth washes prepared by diluting four drops of one of these essential oils in a glass of lukewarm water. Use as gargles and rinses for approximately one to two minutes every two hours.

■ Muscular aches and pains due to over-exertion

These aches may be successfully treated with aromatic baths and relaxing massage treatments with one of the following essential oils: Cypress *(Cupressus sempervirens)*, Ginger *(Zingiber officinalis)*, Rosemary *(Rosmarinus officinalis cineoliferum)*, Scots Pine *(Pinus sylvestris)*, Marjoram *(Origanum majorana)*.

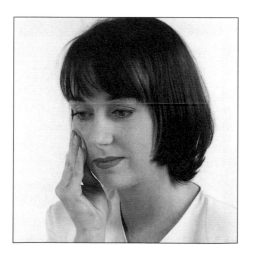

Left: in some cases, acne can be treated effectively with a formulation of aromatherapy oils mixed with a water or Aloe Vera gel base.

AROMATHERAPY FOR BEAUTY

The skin is the largest organ of our body. Amongst its many known functions it has the role of protecting our inner environment, or microcosmos, from the outer surrounding environment, known as the macrocosmos.

The skin ensures thermal regulation through the circulation, by vasoconstriction or closure of capillaries when it is cold, and vasodilation or opening of the capillaries when it is warm.

It also avoids the effects of excessive changes in the weather by increasing sweat to help heat loss from the body.

Certain small molecules, such as those that form the essential oils, are able to penetrate through the layers of the skin and access the various parts of our body via our circulatory and lymphatic systems. Essential oils are perceived increasingly as a necessary integral part of our daily skincare routine. In fact, many well-known cosmetic houses are conducting extensive research into the benefits of essential oils as part of their anti-oxidant skincare products. Aromatherapy skincare is not only nourishing for your skin but also good for your soul and your mind.

Aromatherapy uses essential oils which are specific for your type of skin, age group and/or for the treatment of skin blemishes. The main objectives and functions of a daily skincare routine are: to cleanse, to moisturize, to nourish, to stimulate, and to heal your skin.

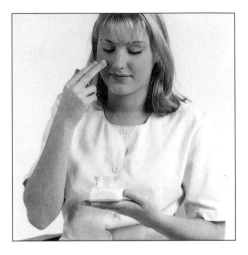

Above: essential oils can be beneficial for all types of skin.

Generally we think of skincare as being only applicable to the face and perhaps to the hands and feet. However, the same ageing processes affect the whole of our skin, so perhaps we should give some further caring thoughts to our entire bodies.

■ Dry or underactive skin

If you have dry or underactive skin your face feels tight, burns easily when exposed to the sun, has a delicate texture, poor elasticity, and has no tone or suppleness and may show some signs of flaking or peeling. The sebaceous glands are producing very little sebum which results in a lack of moisture with an increased premature wrinkling or expression lines. The correct aromatherapy treatment for this type of skin is aimed at improving the circulation via a facial massage, e.g. the routine described in Chapter Three (see page 87). The essential oils beneficial for this type of skin are as follows.

■ **Neroli** *(Citrus aurantium ssp amara)* is anti-inflammatory and increases cell regeneration.

■ **Sandalwood** *(Santalum album)*, is anti-inflammatory, moisturizing and healing.

■ **Rosemary** *(Rosmarinus officinalis verbenone)*, is stimulating, rejuvenating and toning to the skin.

■ Normal skin

If you have normal skin, also known as active skin, your face feels smooth and supple and shows a state of balance and optimum nutrition. The most beneficial oils for this type of skin are:

■ **Fine Lavender** *(Lavandula angustifolia)*, due to its soothing and balancing property.

■ **Geranium** *(Pelargonium odorantissimum)*, which is astringent, moisturizing and rejuvenating.

■ **Patchouli** *(Pogostemum cablin)*, which is a mild antiseptic and skin tonic.

■ **Frankincense** *(Boswellia carterii)*, which is soothing and calming and speeds up cell turnover.

■ Oily or overactive skin

If you have oily or overactive skin your face feels greasy and often has open pores, blackheads and whiteheads. It looks shiny all over and is usually slightly thick. To look after this type of skin choose between the essential oils of:

■ **Ylang Ylang** *(Canaga odorata)*, which is soothing to overactive or oily skin.

■ **Lemon** *(Citrus limonum)*, which may balance the production of sebum while having an anti-infectious effect.

■ **Fine Lavender** *(Lavandula angustifolia)*, for its balancing and healing effects.

■ Sensitive skin

If you have sensitive skin, your face feel very tender and react easily to changes in the weather. It is delicate, generally light in color, and the texture is generally thin. Thus, capillaries can be seen through it. It is prone to couperose, the name given to broken capillaries, mainly on the cheeks and the nose. Generally, it is the type of skin that is most prone to allergies and environmental stresses, such as pollution and extreme temperatures. However, when looked after, it appears to have a porcelain glow and fineness. The essential oils of choice for sensitive skin are:

■ **Neroli** *(Citrus aurantium ssp amara)*, due to its capability to reduce any inflammation and aid cellular regeneration.

■ **German Chamomile** *(Matricaria recutita)*, due to its anti-inflammatory and soothing action on the skin.

■ **Rose** *(Rosa damascena)*, has a hydrating, emolient, and calming action. It also has a mild vasoconstrictive effect which helps to diminish the visibility of surface capillaries.

■ **Frankincense** *(Boswellia carterii)*, has an anti-inflammatory effect and increases the speed of cell turnover, thus preventing the appearance of premature wrinkles.

CHAPTER SIX

AROMATHERAPY FOR INFANTS

Infants always benefit from a gentle aromatherapy massage; it eases minor discomforts, relaxes and balances their entire being, helps them to sleep more peacefully, and strengthens bonding. It is a well-known fact that infants who are frequently stroked and cuddled tend to be happier and more contented.

In many parts of the world, infant massage techniques are passed on from generation to generation, from the grandmother to the new mother. Stroking, stretching and spreading the special moisturizing oils, and gently mobilizing the infant's body are considered essential for the new child's developmental needs and his bonding with his mother and father.

Infant massage can be started from the first week after birth. You can commence the massage by gently massaging your baby's skin with a cold-pressed Sweet Almond oil or Peach kernel oil. Essential oils should not be used in infant massage until the baby is at least six months old. At this time a 0.5% dilution of essential oil of Fine Lavender (*Lavandula angustifolia*) may be used in the massage blend once a week. This oil will help to improve the baby's natural resistance to infections.

MASSAGE GUIDELINES

■ You can massage your baby daily for a period of 20 to 30 minutes. A good time is before meals, as you should not interfere with the digestive processes.

■ Ensure that the room where you wish to perform the massage is warm, that there are no drafts, violent noises, or any other disturbance which may startle your baby and intrude on this quiet bonding time on your own with him.

■ The length of time spent in the massage is not rigid but may vary and be adjusted according to your baby's age. As the baby grows, he may want to help and join in, wriggle and turn as he enjoys being massaged.

■ The best way to massage your baby is to place him on your stretched-out legs, while you either sit on the floor, leaning against a wall if this feels more comfortable, or on a hard bed in the same position. The baby's head should rest on your knees and his feet should be pointing to your chest.

■ Have two warm towels close at hand in case you need to cover the baby.

■ Do not use essential oils on young babies; use Sweet Almond oil instead.

INFANT MASSAGE

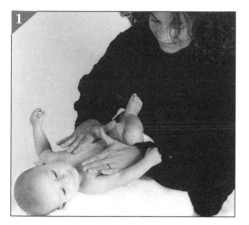
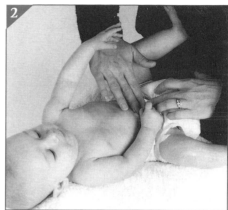
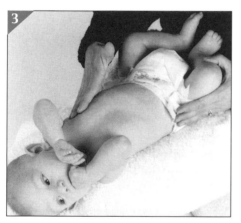
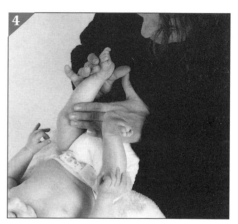

1 With stroking light effleurage, spread the massage oil on the front of the baby's body. Remember to pour the oil on your cupped hand first, so that when it reaches the baby it has warmed up to body temperature and feels comforting. Work toward the heart in the center of the chest to follow and encourage the normal flow of blood.

2 Very gently in a clockwise direction, massage the abdomen. First, in a small circle around the navel, then in a larger circle around the outer edges of the abdomen.

3 Start on the lower right and work upward toward the rib cage, then across to the left rib cage and downward on the left-hand side. This should be a continuous circular clockwise movement.

4 With one hand, hold your baby's left foot and stroke it gently, then stroke and gently squeeze in an upward movement until you reach the groin. Glide back down to the foot and repeat several times.

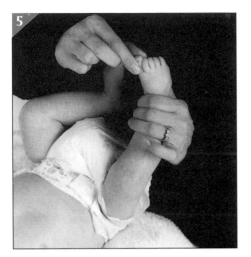

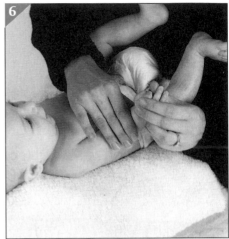

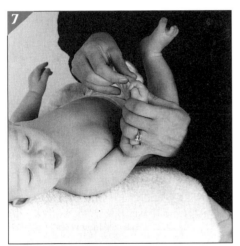

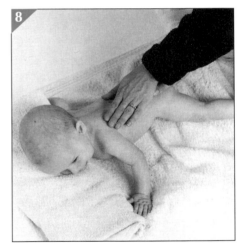

5 Hold the foot and, with your thumb, massage the sole and finish by gently stretching and rotating each toe between your thumb and index finger. Repeat the sequence on the left lower limb.

6 In your hand, hold your baby's right hand and slightly stretch the upper limb, then lightly squeeze and stroke upward toward the armpit until you reach it. Then glide back to the baby's hand and repeat several times.

7 Return to the hand and gently open the grip of the palm and work on each finger, rotating it gently between your own thumb and index finger. Repeat with the right upper limb.

8 Turn the baby over and position him lying comfortably on his tummy. Stroke your baby's back from the feet to the shoulders to apply and spread the oil.

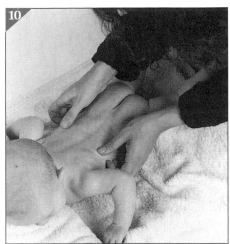

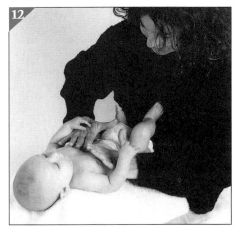

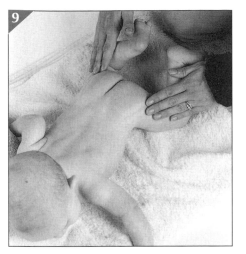

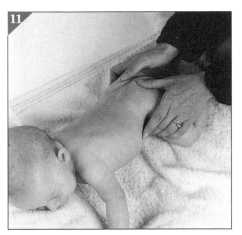

9 Then turn your hands outward and glide down the sides until you reach the toes. Repeat several times.

10 Starting at the baby's bottom, place one hand on each side and work your way up to the shoulders with wringing motions. Then work your way down again, crossing your hands repeatedly from one side to the other. Repeat several times.

11 Cup one hand around the baby's bottom and place your other hand on the back of the neck. Glide the upper hand firmly down the back to meet the lower hand. Stroke around the buttocks and gently press them together.

12 Now repeat the upward stroking movements, gradually making the strokes slower and longer to relax the baby completely and get him ready for sleep. At the end of the massage, very gently turn your baby over, wrap him in a soft blanket and give him a big cuddle.

CHAPTER SEVEN

AROMATHERAPY FOR LOVERS AND DREAMERS

It has long been known and established that some essential oils can act as aphrodisiacs and help to create the appropriate mood for loving and dreaming. Correctly used, aromatherapy may be very beneficial if you are suffering from stress and tension, which can prevent you relaxing and enjoying tender and dreamy moments with your loved one.

CREATING A SENSUOUS MOOD

To create a very romantic and sensual environment, choose a blend of three of

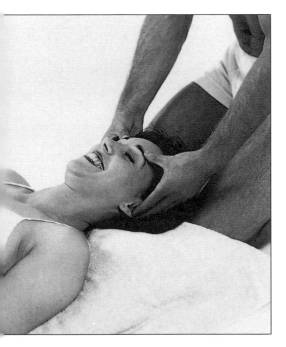

your favorite oils, e.g. four drops of Sandalwood (*Santalum album*), four drops of Rose (*Rosa damascena*), and four drops of Ylang Ylang (*Canaga odorata*). Blend the essential oils with 20ml of your favorite base oil—a very luxurious one consists of equal parts of Rosehip seed and Jojoba. This gives your skin extra nourishment and a healthy glow.

You may also add one of your chosen oils to your room diffuser, so that the scent permeates the whole area. I do not recommend using another aroma in the room as this may spoil the final desired effect. As for any other type of massage, you must ensure that the room is kept pleasantly warm.

You may use any of the relaxing or stimulating massage techniques described previously in this book if you wish, but it is always more exciting to explore each other's bodies and find your own special favorite areas and massage techniques. Leave things to develop gradually, and allow yourself and your partner to play, tease, excite and awaken each other's bodies—use your imagination. Make sure

Left: a relaxing and sensuous massage with aromatic essential oils can enhance your relationship.

there are no time constraints or unwanted interruptions. When you finish the massage you may wish to take an aromatic bath together, or have a candlelit dinner just for the two of you.

We all know that when it comes to day dreaming we are able to let our fantasy guide our steps. In this case, you should allow your intuition to remember and recreate that elusive fragrance or blend of essential oils which has been at the back of your mind for so many years. The descriptions of the psychological and emotional aspects of each essential oil in Chapter Two should help you in your quest. Remember that you are the dreamer and the lover, and only you and your partner are able to make your intimate moments together a precious time to remember for ever and ever.

ROMANTIC OIL FORMULATIONS

Some tested essential oil formulations you may find useful are the following. Remember that they will all require a base oil.

APHRODITE

Essential oil of Rose	
(Rosa damascena)	2 drops
Essential oil of Frankincense	
(Boswellia carterii)	3 drops
Essential oil of Ginger	
(Zingiber officinalis)	2 drops
Essential oil of Rosewood	
(Aniba rosaeodora var amazonica)	3 drops

APOLLO

Essential oil of Vetiver	
(Vetiveria zizanoides)	1 drop
Essential oil of Eucalyptus C.	
(Eucalyptus citriodora)	3 drops
Essential oil of Sandalwood	
(Santalum album)	3 drops
Essential oil of Patchouli	
(Pogostemon cablin)	1 drop
Essential oil of Rose	
(Rosa damascena)	2 drops

ZEUS

Essential oil of Frankincense	
(Boswellia carterii)	2 drops
Essential oil of Sandalwood	
(Santalum album)	3 drops
Essential oil of Geranium	
(Pelargonium odorantissimum)	3 drops
Essential oil of Bergamot	
(Citrus bergamia)	2 drops
Essential oil of Neroli	
(Citrus aurantium ssp amara)	4 drops

BEATRIZ

Essential oil of Rose	
(Rosa damascena)	4 drops
Essential oil of Neroli	
(Citrus aurantium ssp amara)	3 drops
Essential oil of Chamomile Moroccan	
(Ormenis mixta)	2 drops
Essential oil of Petitgrain	
(Citrus aurantium ssp amara)	3 drops
Essential oil of Lemon	
(Citrus limonum)	3 drops

USEFUL ADDRESSES

GETTING PROFESSIONAL HELP

It is advisable to visit a qualified clinical aromatherapy practitioner when seeking professional help. A professional aromatherapy practitioner is not only able to identify your personal needs through a lengthy consultation but also to prepare a specific formulation for you as an individual suffering from a number of complaints, and provide specialized and skilled treatment techniques.

A professional aromatherapy practitioner will be a member of a professional body which requires its members to abide by its codes of ethics and standards, and gets regular updates on any new research and developments related to safe professional clinical practice. The professional bodies provide an individual practitioner with proper insurance cover. This means that a member of the public who visits an aromatherapist may do so with the full confidence of knowing that the practitioner has the adequate and appropriate level of training, and the necessary knowledge and skill that enable them to look after their clients' health needs.

Always ask to see your practitioner's qualifications at the time of your first consultation. A bona fide professional will never object to this and will be only too eager to let you see them. When looking for a practitioner in your area, it is advisable to contact any of the professional organizations listed below. They will be able to help and advise you.

UNITED STATES

AROMATHERAPY

National Association for Holistic Aromatherapy
219 Carl Street
San Francisco
CA 94117–3804
Tel: (415) 564–6785

MASSAGE

American Massage Therapy Association
820 Davis Street
Suite 100
Evanston
IL 60201–4444
Tel: (708) 864–0123

International Association of Infant Massage
2350 Bowen Road
Elma
NY 14059
Tel: (800) 248–5432

UNITED KINGDOM

The Institute for Complementary Medicine
Unit 15
Tavern Quay
Commercial Centre
Rope Street
London SE16 1TX
Tel: 0171 237 5165

For information on registered practitioners in

most forms of
Complementary Medicine,
you should contact:
The British Register of
Complementary
Practitioners
P.O. Box 194
London
SE16 1QZ
Tel/fax: 0171 237 5175

International Federation
of Aromatherapists
Stamford House
2–4 Chiswick High Road
London
W4 1TH

Register of Qualified
Aromatherapists
P.O. Box 6941

London N8 9HF

International Society of
Professional
Aromatherapists
ISPA House
82 Ashby Road
Hinckley, Leicestershire
LE10 1SF

Guild of Complementary
Practitioners
Alpha House
High Street
Crawthorne
Berkshire
RG45 7AD

Aromatherapy
Organisations Council
3 Latymer Close

Baybrooke
Market Harborough,
Leicestershire
LE16 8LN

AUSTRALIA

International Federation
of Aromatherapists
(Australian branch) Inc.
5 Uren Place
Kambahact 2902
Australia
Tel/fax: Australia 06 231
0707

FURTHER READING

Bradford, Nicky, *The Well Woman's Self Help Directory*
Bradford, Nicky, *Men's Health Matters*
Bradford, Nicky, *Hamlyn's Encyclopedia of Complementary Medicine*
Davis, P., *The A to Z of Aromatherapy*
Franchomme, P., and Penouel, D., *L'Aromatherapie Exactement*
Grayson, Jane, *The Fragrant Year*
Lawrence, Brian, *Essential Oils*

Lunny, Dr. V., *I.F.A. Times Articles*
M. Maury, *The Secret of Life and Youth*
Price, S., *Practical Aromatherapy*
Tisserand, R., *Aromatherapy for Everyone*
Valnet, Dr. J., *Aromatherapie*
Werner, Monica, *Aromatherapie*
Werner, Monica, *Sanfte Massage*
Worwood, V.A., *The Fragrant Pharmacy*
Worwood, V.A., *The Fragrant Mind*